STEPPING STONES

STONES

— TO —

Recovery ®

For Women

Experience the miracle of 12 Step Recovery

Copyright © 1989 by Glen Abbey Books, Inc.

Published by Glen Abbey Books, Inc.

Printed in the United States of America
Cover design by Graphiti, Inc., Seattle, Washington

Library of Congress Cataloging in Publication Data

Stepping stones to recovery for women.
        p.   cm.
    ISBN 0-934125-15-5 : $6.95
    1. Alcoholics--Rehabilitation. 2. Women--Alco-
hol use. 3. Women--Religious life.
HV5278.S74   1989
362.29'286'082--dc20   89-17751
                                             CIP

The following have given permission to use reprints of: (1) "Co-
dependency: An Intimacy Dilemma," by Sondra Smalley, reprinted
by permission of the author; (2) "I Don't Go to Meetings Anymore,"
reprinted by permission of A.A. Grapevine, Inc.

Disclaimer: The publication of this volume does not imply affili-
ation with nor approval or endorsement from Alcoholics Anonymous World Services, Inc.

10 9 8 7 6 5 4 3 2

This Book Is Dedicated

To

SPONSORS

CONTENTS

GUIDE FOR DAILY READING

GUIDE FOR DAILY READING

GUIDE FOR DAILY READING

GUIDE FOR DAILY READING

PREFACE

The articles, poems and slogans in this anthology are for all of us who are recovering from our addiction in one of the Twelve-Step Fellowships. I would like to thank the following individuals for their help in the preparation of this book: Susan Jensen, Linda McClelland, Michelle Ogata, and Bill Pittman.

Special thanks to all those who have contributed articles for this book, including the individuals who wish to remain anonymous, and to the following:

Ann	Harriett B.	M.B.
Betty P.	Helen S.	Marilyn D.
Brenda T.	Jeanne V. T.	Mary Lou A.
Carol S.	Jeneane C.	Mimi M.
D.F.	Jenny C.	Nina W.
Debbie L.	Julie M.	P.R.
Dorothy B.	Karen S.	Patti
Dot F.	Kathlee M.	Robin R.
Edna	Kathy K.	Sheila D.
Esther G.	Linda L. D.	Sheree S.
	Liz B.	Vickie M.

Mary B., Editor

1. DROP THE ROCK
(Character defects)

Seems there was this group of 12 Step members taking a boat ride to this island called SERENITY, and they were truly a happy bunch of people. As the boat pulled away from the dock, a few on board noticed Mary running down the street trying to catch up with the boat. One said, "Darn, she's missed the boat." Another said, "Maybe not. Come on, Mary! Jump in the water! Swim! Swim! You can make it! You can catch up with us!"

So Mary jumped into the water and started to swim for all she was worth. She swam for quite a while, and then started to sink. The members on board, now all aware that Mary was struggling, shouted, "Come on, Mary! Don't give up! Drop the rock!" With that encouragement, Mary started swimming again, only to start sinking again shortly afterward. She was going under when she heard all those voices shouting to her, "Mary, drop the rock! Let go, and drop the rock!"

Mary was vaguely aware of something around her neck, but she couldn't quite figure out what it was. Once more, she gathered her strength and started swimming. She was doing quite well, even gaining a little on the boat, but then she felt this heaviness pulling her under again. She saw all those people on the boat holding out their hands and hollering for her to keep swimming and shouting, "Don't be an idiot, Mary! Drop the rock!"

Then she understood, when she was going down for the third time. This thing around her neck, *this* was why she kept sinking when she really *wanted* to catch the boat. This thing was the "rock" they were all shouting about: resentments, fear, dishonesty, self-pity, intolerance and anger, just some of the things her "rock" was made of. "Get rid of the rock," she told herself. "Now! Get rid of it!"

So Mary managed to stay afloat long enough to untangle a few of the strings holding that rock around her neck, realizing as she did that her load was easing up; and then, with another burst of energy, she Let Go. She tore the other strings off and Dropped the Rock.

Once free of the rock, she was amazed how easy it was to swim, and she soon caught up with the boat. Those on board were cheering for her and applauding and telling her how great she was, and how it was so good having her with them again, and how now we can get on with our boat ride and have a nice time.

Mary felt great and was just about to indulge in a little rest and relaxation when she glanced back to shore. There, a ways back, she thought she saw something bobbing in the water, so she pointed it out to some others. Sure enough, someone was trying to catch the boat, swimming for dear life but not making much headway. In fact, it looked like they were going under.

Mary looked around and saw the concern on the faces of the other members. She was the first to lean over the rail and shout, "Hey, friend! Drop the Rock!"

2.   MOMENTS OF CLARITY
(Gratitude)

My sponsor asked me to slow down and write about gratitude, and I immediately went into a panic. I am one of those who rarely is aware of being grateful. Until I came into this program, the terms being "grateful" and "feeling gratitude" were totally alien to me. If I have ever achieved a state of perfectionism, it is in the area of negativity.

It is now the day before I am to turn this in, and after much pondering:

I am not happy that my ex-landlord is one of "them" and made it necessary for me to move this past month; but I am grateful that he motivated me into moving out of a 9-year rut and I now have a beautiful apartment.

I am not happy that I didn't get the amount of raise that I felt I should; but I am grateful that it is sufficient to cover the extra expense of my new apartment.

I am not happy that I had to give away one of my cats; but I am grateful that one of my best friends took her and I know the cat has a good home.

I am not happy that I've been in a great deal of physical pain lately; but I am grateful that it is nothing serious and can be easily remedied.

I am not happy that my daughter is having serious problems and has had to manipulate her family into a geographic; but I am grateful that it brought her from the east coast to southern California.

I am not happy that my niece is into drugs; but I am grateful that she has entered into a drug rehab program.

Since I got started, I could go on ad infinitum.

Just as I thought I had to like something to accept it, I guess I thought something had to make me happy before I could be grateful.

I thank God for this Program, and I thank this Program for these moments of clarity.

3.   SELF-KNOWLEDGE ISN'T ENOUGH
(Steps 6, 7, 8 and 9)

Recently I was perusing ahead in my daily meditation book when I came upon a quote by Martha

Roth which piqued my curiosity. "Insight is cheap," she said. My first reaction was "Gee, I don't agree with her. We in recovery place high value on insight. After all, it's our insight regarding the problem of addiction which makes us particularly helpful to 'the person who still suffers,'" but, as I read the short essay following the quote, I began to see Ms. Roth's point.

She talked about people who analyze themselves to death. They know just exactly what makes them do the things they do: the tyrannical mothers, the abusive husbands, the poverty they were raised in or the childhood of extreme indulgence, ad nauseum.

They have great insight; but instead of using that insight as a means to develop new and, hopefully, better behavior, they use it as a reason to continue with old, destructive behavior. They are not willing to go through the pain it takes to change, even though the pain of staying the same is killing them.

They are victims. The list of people who've done them wrong is long, and the list of those people whose expectations they cannot live up to is even longer. They cling to their character defects with alarming tenacity, all the while pleading a "Mommy Dearest" or "Burning Bed" defense.

In fact, they don't see their poor behavior as character defects at all, but more like genetic anomalies, such as bowlegs or thin hair, or the permanent result of improper socialization by parents who did the best job they could, but nevertheless did a crappy job.

"Admitting that they may be somewhat at fault, they are sure others are more to blame," therefore, instead of asking God to remove any defects of character, they secretly curse God for dealing them such a lousy hand.

They are good at working with newcomers, especially if the newcomer is attractive and a member of the opposite sex (or same sex, if they are so inclined). The problem here is that all they want to do is talk about themselves and all the newcomer wants to do is talk about herself, so these liaisons rarely last more than a few days or weeks before they bore each other to the brink of suicide.

While they rarely balk at Steps 4 and 5 because those steps give them the opportunity once again to dwell on their most beloved topic, themselves, they seem to get stuck at this point and gloss over or ignore completely those steps in the program which are vital to emotional and spiritual recovery: Steps 6, 7, 8 and 9.

And, without emotional and spiritual recovery, you don't have much. You have abstinence, and you may not even have that for very long.

4. LEARN TO LOVE ONE ANOTHER
(Overcoming a dysfunctional home)

When I first came to the Fellowship, I did not know how to love. I still don't! All I know is that what I'm doing feels pretty good. Externally, the evidence is there; internally, I am not sure whether I am feeling the way the songwriters say I should, but it will have to do. I don't know any better.

If love is blind, so is the knowledge of love. I "love" eating an orange, but I don't know whether I'm enjoying it any more or less than you are. We can't experience each other's sensations.

If I've learned to love in recovery, it's been by not trying to learn to love at all, but by trying to do something else. Like many other members I've heard, I come from a background deficient not only in love, but in the fundamental intimacies enjoyed in most families.

When I came into the program, I was told that if I wanted to recover, I would have to learn to love; that in order to learn to love anyone else, I would have to learn to love myself. I didn't know what the heck they were talking about.

They told me that the first thing I had to do, as with so many of my other attitudes, was get rid of the physical thinking -- love is love, not lust. It was a relief to me, after some study, to come to the conclusion that love does not really exist in itself; it is a "description of something else." But what?

When I posed this earthshaking question to my fellow members, I was told, "Keep coming to meetings, work the Program and try to help others do the same thing. And if you feel like talking, here's my number. Call me anytime."

I compared this response to that of a local running club, of which I am a member. Nice people, all of them. Friendly, helpful and mutually supportive in our common efforts to improve our physical being. But deeply caring, sharing, loving? No. And that's the big difference.

My home group is a gathering of sharing, caring, loving people. More important, they love each other as distinct individuals, not as members of a group. Why? Because they need each other, and they know it. Further, they are willing to admit it out loud. To love is to acknowledge an interrelationship, and therein is psychic strength.

Through the Twelve Steps, I was shown how to sweep aside the primacy of concern with self, to discard the selfishness and arrogance that stood in the way. All these were obstacles to love; and as I began to learn to turn my life and will over to God as I understood Him, the faint glimmerings of humility began to appear.

And with this came, finally, the spiritual

awakening that was the beginning, for the first time in my life, of that unique experience we inadequately call love. It was not the "I want everyone to love me and I'll do anything to get it" love. It was simply "I love you," without reservation, qualification, or expectation. Love can be offered with a smile.

In recovery, I have learned that we are all born with a single set of instructions: to love one another. Our success in this world depends totally on how well we follow those instructions.

5. TIME TO CHANGE
(Too busy to change?)

Many 12 Step members, in recovery for some length of time, often encounter situations or circumstances in their lives that overwhelm them to the extent that a period of time is needed for self-examination, a renewed effort in working the 12 Steps, a greater need for prayer, attending more meetings, and relying heavily on the Fellowship and their sponsor's advice.

The emotional pain can be acute because we tell ourselves we should be further along or more well than what we actually are. And, if we are being honest, the pain and fear of rejection by our fellow members makes an honest disclosure of our present difficulties a hard task. But truly we must tell it like it is to remain sane and stay in recovery.

My sponsor and my own experiences are teaching me that this is normal and that if I take the right attitude, it can be a time of personal healing and growth. It is difficult to see the people you have been sponsoring start to turn away. It is difficult to realize you sometimes have nothing to share at your meetings and that your interest in your commitments is waning, your heart isn't in it, so to speak.

My sponsor told me she went through two years of this. She did not stop going to meetings or working the 12 Steps. She simply took the time to receive what she needed to hear or do to get well for herself. She laid aside the principle of giving of yourself for just a time and told me this was difficult for her to do. She assured me that after she had devoted this time to straightening out her personal problems, she was a much stronger person for it and could get back into helping others, no longer feeling like she couldn't give away something she didn't have.

There should be no shame in admitting we don't have it all together at times. True, there is our pride and ego to overcome in making this disclosure to others. But the Program teaches me this is humility, and by so humbling myself I grow in the sunlight of the Spirit. After all, didn't I make this very disclosure known to you all when I first came through the door and took my First Step?

6. THE THREE ANSWERS TO PRAYER
(Steps 3, 7, and 11)

I believe there are three answers to prayer: YES, NO and WAIT.

Many times I do not hear those answers because I am not listening. Sometimes I do not respond out of ignorance. After many years of diligently seeking conscious contact with God, I am finally learning to pay attention.

When my Higher Power says YES to a prayer, I often find that the next thing I need is courage to take the action. Generally, I know what to do but I am held back by fear, which I understand to be the opposite of faith.

When I hear NO, I am sustained by God's infinite wisdom. Today I believe God knows what is best for me.

The answer, WAIT, calls for patience, a new quality in my life that was missing in the past when I compulsively sought instant gratification through my addictions.

I am grateful for the Twelve Steps, which have taught me to listen for God's answers whether it be through the first Three Steps, which help me achieve abstinence; Steps Four through Nine, the prerequisites for recovery; or Steps Ten through Twelve, the maintenance mantle of protection.

I find special solace in Steps Three, Seven and Eleven, the quiet havens where I find God's answers to my prayers: YES, NO and WAIT.

7.   FIRST YEAR ANNIVERSARY

It is now a year since I came to the Fellowship. The first six months, my body came; and the next six months my head was to come and make me whole.

With my whole self now, I can work with and at my recovery, which is a very gradual process and goes along at a comfortable pace.

I make a new conquest each day, whether physical, emotional, or spiritual. Yes, a day at a time I am getting better.

My walk through the 12 Steps has been good, bad, happy, and sad. All upsets and all rewards are all due to the Fellowship, my group, and hard honest work on my part.

It's a complete wonder that I am in recovery today, never mind writing about gratitude. I thank God and all his children in and out of the Fellowship for lending the support and comfort when I need it. Need is in the present as I will always want and need my fellow human beings.

8.   UNKNOWN LESS
        FRIGHTENING NOW
        (Overcoming fear)

As I approached my life in this 12 Step Program, my greatest fear was leaving behind the only life I had ever known. It was filled with fear, loneliness and self-centeredness. It's hard to believe that I wanted so desperately to hold on to such a life, but the truth of the matter is, it was familiar and in a strange way, very comfortable. The old Chinese proverb says, "I would rather live with the seven dragons I know than the one strange dragon I don't know."

The changes I was so afraid of have become comfortable today. If I have anything to say to the newcomer today it is, "Our Fellowship began from the very start to make the unknown less frightening than the known." It helped me come from a person who was completely self-centered to a person who can see a Power greater than myself, from a person who was so dominated by fear to a place where I'm not so often in fear and anxiety and to where I am at a point of spending much of my time with a measure of peace. I used to think the world was a terrifying place, a place I tried so hard to get out of. Now I find it a beautiful place with peace and contentment in recovery that far exceeds my expectations.

Please don't misunderstand the fact that I still

have some pretty rough times. With the changes that have taken place they are certainly there; but through this Program I have come full circle in my spiritual life, and underneath it all, I know, are God's everlasting arms.

As it says in A.A.'s Big Book, *"Half measures availed us nothing. We asked His protection and care with complete abandon."* Those words have convinced me I must take this Program pretty seriously, not to just patch or tidy things up a little, but I need to give this Program my daily attention, holding nothing back; and the funny thing is, the more I love and work this Program, the more guarantees I have that I will have more of God's love and goodness in my life.

I know today I am somebody. The 12 Steps have helped me to feel good enough about myself to know *I do count* in God's plans. For me, that's real progress.

9.   TWELVE STEPS FOR A SPONSOR

1.   I will not help you stay and wallow in limbo.
2.   I will help you grow, to become more productive, by your own definition.
3.   I will help you become more autonomous,

more loving of yourself, more free to continue
becoming the authority of your own living.

4.   I cannot give you dreams or "fix you up,"
simply because I cannot.

5.   I cannot give you growth, or grow for you.
You must grow yourself, by facing reality,
grim as it may be at times.

6.   I cannot take away your loneliness or pain.

7.   I cannot sense your world for you, evaluate
your goals, or tell you what is best for you in
your world; you have your own world.

8.   I cannot convince you of the crucial choice of
choosing the scary uncertainty of growing
over the safe misery of not growing.

9.   I want to be with you and know you as a rich
and growing friend, yet I cannot get close to
you when you choose not to grow.

10.   When I begin to care for you out of pity, when
I begin to lose trust in you, then I am toxic, bad
and inhibiting for you, and you for me.

11.   You must know my help is conditional. I will
be with you, hang in there with you, as long as
I continue to get even the slightest hints that
you are trying to grow.

12.   If you can accept all of this, then perhaps we
can help each other to become what God
meant us to be: mature adults, leaving child-
ishness forever to little children.

10. THE VALUE OF FUNDAMENTALS
(Guidelines for meetings)

We are often told, when we get disgusted with meetings and tired of hearing the talk of others in the group, to look within ourselves, that probably there is something wrong with our thinking, rather than that the group is wrong.

Group meetings do tend to stagnate at times, and the group can examine its group conscience just as the individual must on many occasions. Hilarious antics of pre-recovery days are screamingly funny; psychiatric reactions from our addiction are interesting; arguments on religion are worthwhile; service discussions have their place. But they don't fit into 12-Step meetings.

Our primary purpose is to get into recovery and stay in recovery. We do this through our 12 Steps. Deviate for long from this fundamental course of action and experience shows that group unrest starts to grow.

The longer one is in a 12-Step fellowship, the more one appreciates the value of fundamentals. No finer meeting can be enjoyed than that devoted to basic 12-Step principles.

11. HAVING FAITH
(Step 2)

I really never believed in anything before I got to the Program. I didn't believe in God, other people, and especially, I didn't believe in myself nor my ability to recover. Gradually, just by sitting in meetings and hearing other members talk about being abstinent for a few days or several years, I came to believe that I too, with the help of the 12 Steps, could stay abstinent. This Fellowship truly was the first thing I can remember having faith in; and that faith saved my life. Before the 12 Steps, my life seemed empty, devoid of meaning. Faith has given my life meaning and direction. Besides faith in this Fellowship and the 12 Steps, I now believe in God and many other things. I can't imagine going back to my old way of life, full of fear and void of faith.

To me, faith is like gratitude. It's a gift from my Higher Power and like any other gift, it is not something to which I am entitled. If I abuse it and don't practice the principles of the Program, I can lose it as well as my recovery. That's one of the great benefits I have received from the Fellowship and the 12 Steps. I can now benefit from others' experience and not have to learn everything the hard way.

Faith has really transformed my life. It is the essence of the Second Step, and without it, I would not have kept coming back.

12.   GOD'S PLAN FOR ME

God has a plan for me. It is hidden within me, just as the oak is hidden within the acorn or the rose within the bud. As I yield myself more fully to God, His Plan expresses itself more perfectly through me. I can tell when I am in tune with it, for then my mind and my heart are filled with a deep inner peace. This peace fills me with a sense of security, with joy, and a desire to take the Steps that are a part of the Plan.

God's Plan for me is a perfect part of a larger Plan. It is designed for the good of all and not for me alone. It is a many-sided Plan and reaches out through all the people I meet. All the events and people who come into my life are instruments of the unfolding of this Plan.

God has chosen those people He wants me to know, to love and to serve. We are continually being drawn to one another in ways that are not coincidental. I pray that I may become a better instrument to love and to serve and that I may become more worthy to receive the love and service of others.

I ask the Father within me for only those things which He wants me to have. I know that these benefits will come to me at the right time and in the right way. This inner knowing frees my mind and heart from fear, greed, jealousy, anger and resentment. It gives me courage and faith to do those things which I feel are mine to do. I no longer look with envy at what others are receiving. Therefore, I do not cut myself off from God, the giver of all good things.

God's gifts to me can be many times greater than I am now receiving. I pray that I may increase my capacity to give, for I can give only as I receive and receive only as I give.

I believe that when I cannot do those things I desire to do, it is because God has closed one door only to leave ajar a better and larger door. If I do not see the door just ahead, it is because I have not seen, heard, or obeyed God's guidance. It is then that God uses the trouble of seeming failure which may result to help me face myself and see the new opportunity before me.

The real purpose of my life is to find God within my own mind and heart and to help others. I thank my Father for each experience which helps me to surrender my will to His will. For only as I lose myself in the consciousness of His Great Presence can His Plan for my life be fulfilled.

13.   MAKING THE RIGHT CHOICE

When I got up this morning, I was faced with the same choice that I face every day of my life. Is the day going to be a *bore* and a *chore* or will it be an adventure? Needless to say, in my life I haven't always made the right choice at the right moment; and in the world of reality there are tragedies and events beyond our control. But I believe that with the tools the Fellowship has given me I do have a choice. In fact, if I truly start my day by asking "His protection and care with complete abandon" and then just go on out and be myself, then I have a right to *expect* the day to be an adventure; and you know what? It happens!

At times in my life I have allowed others to make that choice for me; and certainly, when I was using, there was no possibility of choice. So I am forced to accept the one fact that I ran from all of my life. I AM RESPONSIBLE. Even God cannot make that choice for me. Granted, it is helpful to be surrounded by good friends and loved ones. But it is not *required*. I have learned to have a great day alone with God if I so choose. I love our Third Step prayer in the Big Book which says "relieve me of the bondage of Self." I usually learn things the hard way, and today I know by my own long and painful experience that it really is *that simple*.

14.   I'M NOT ALONE ANYMORE

Tonight, I entered the meeting, looked around, thought, "What the hell am I doing here? They're all too young here." Then I began to cry, stealthily, secretively, privately. In the midst of love, I chose to sit in loneliness. I thought about asking Brian to hug me.

Linda came in with Dave; and I thought of going over and asking for a hug, even though the readings had begun. I didn't. I sat and hid my tears and wondered what I was doing in this particular meeting at this particular time.

Thank God for the Fellowship. Tonight I listened to a woman who has lost two intimate relationships to death in the last three years. Suddenly I knew I was in the right meeting, after all. No one is too young to have known loss. I was in the right meeting after all. When it came my turn to speak, I knew I would be understood. Tonight, after I was honest with myself and with the group about how scared I was to cry, even after all these years on the Program, and how scared I was to ask for hugs when I needed them, I received so many hugs after the meeting that I felt like a queen.

Thank God for the Fellowship. I went with so much pain that I didn't know if I was going to be able to stop crying. After the meeting, I am back into today, again accepting the death of my lovely son. And, yes, the task I am engaged in *is* hard. But with God's help, I am equal to it. I want to be sure to thank people who went out of their way to say, "I love you. I'm sorry you hurt. I'm here if you need me; you are not alone." I have waited sixteen months to start the process because I wasn't ready before. I knew I wasn't able to handle the extra pain. But now I *can* handle it. With God's help and because I am a part of the Fellowship, I can now write my appreciations for the loving words

I received. It's time.

It's so paradoxical: I am alone; I am not alone. These are equal truths. Alone was I born; alone will I die; yet I am not alone. I demand that God Be. I need to believe that the Spirit survives and that survival has something to do with what we call "God," the force that we are all part of: the planets, the suns, the flowers, the gases that swirl in a comet's tail, and we finite beings on this little ball that whirls in orderly fashion in its space. So I thank God, without concern for His/Her/Its shape or form. The Fellowship has proven the existence of Spirit to me. Since love exists, God exists.

15.   ONLY THREE THINGS TO CHANGE

When I first came into the Fellowship, I thought all I needed to do was to stay abstinent. Then I began hearing about needing to change other aspects of my life, and I didn't like it a bit. My sponsor realized that I was very resistant to change; and when I began discussing it with her, instead of giving me a long list of things I would need to change, she said not to worry as there were only three things a newcomer needed to change.

I was relieved to hear that and said I could handle just three things and asked what they were, ready to get at it. My sponsor said, "Everything you say, everything you think, and everything you do." Then she smiled. I didn't. I do now.

16.   H.O.W.
(Honest, Openminded and Willing)

I would like to share something that has freed me from bondage of self and allowed me to know serenity. It is something that I have heard time and time again in meetings, but didn't really pay much attention to unless I was absolutely dying inside.

When I was so miserable inside myself (even in recovery) that I couldn't stand to live in my own skin, when suicide became an option, I would finally turn to my Higher Power. I would get some relief from the pain. But for some reason, after I began to feel better, and I always did, I turned back to Self and inevitably, I ended up in misery again.

What was it that kept me from continuing on that spiritual path? Some say it is because I am an addict; and I am, by virtue of that fact, selfish and self-centered by nature. But did I listen? Nope! I had to learn it by experience, my own experience.

I am a great one for taking surveys. I got into the Program and began immediately asking people how they "did it"! What did they do to not only stay abstinent but live a happy life? That's what I wanted for me.

Every one of the people I talked to are on an active and ongoing "spiritual path" of some kind. Some go to church regularly; some don't. Some meditate and pray a lot; some read pages 85, 86, 87 and 88 in the Big Book every day; some do other things. But they all continue an active and ongoing search for information relating to their own Higher Power. They are all Honest, Openminded and Willing.

Why have I ignored this cliche in the past? I don't know. But I do know that since I have kept up my own ongoing spiritual journey, my life has improved. My world could be crumbling around me (and it has) and it doesn't seem to affect my serenity level. It only inspires me to do more.

I took an inventory on all this, and I found that my spiritual quest was very sporadic. When I put it down for a while, I was miserable. When it became the most important thing in my life and the most constant thing in my life, I became happier.

The Fellowship is a huge part of my spiritual path, because it not only offers me new information and understanding, but it also allows me to share it with others.

17.   IS THIS FOR REAL?
(Sharing love and kindness)

When they first come into our Program, many

newcomers are hesitant about spreading love and friendship. They pull back from the hugging, the laughter and the smiles.

Some of them still believe the twisted truths they grew up with, the things their parents pointed out: "You only have so much love; don't waste it; don't give it away to anyone who comes along."

For those people, giving freely is a chore. They are convinced, in their own way, there is only so much love to give and, once it is used up, the well of kindness and love runs dry forever.

In almost any shopping mall, in many flower shops, and in some department stores today you'll find one or more small cascading waterfalls. These tiny pieces of nature are usually recreated with man-made rocks. The soft gurgle of a babbling brook and a tiny waterfall continues endlessly.

The fact is, the amount of water used in these waterfall displays is usually limited and, in some instances, quite small, usually only a few gallons.

The secret of how a gallon or so of water can power an endless cascade of bubbling, spring-like water is a recirculating pump. The same water falls to the reflecting pool bottom of the display and is re-pumped back to the top to begin descending all over again.

So it is with love and kindness. In our Fellowship, a small touch, a smile, a fleeting touch of a friendly hand primes the pump of recirculating love.

The shared knowledge that we all suffer from the same addiction, we all carry the same problems and failures, the same delights and successes, keeps the recirculating pump of endless love and laughter always in motion.

The more you give, the more you get as you help newcomers to realize happiness is a choice, honesty is a habit, and love freely given is a divine gift that never grows smaller with use, but one that grows stronger with every smile, strengthening the invisible umbilical cord of addiction that ties us all, one to the other.

18. "WOE IS ME!"
(Keeping the faith)

I've never been very good at making out a gratitude list, even though my sponsor has suggested it. At times I get lost in the worries of this world--money, prestige, possessions, appearances, etc. I worry about my jalopy car not making it (it has over 100,000 miles on it). I worry about paying the electric bill and about supplying my son with $1.50 a day for lunch money. Sometimes I feel sorry for myself because I wear mostly hand-me-down clothes. I have a granddaughter who is 1-1/2 years old, and I've never seen her. WOE IS ME!

Isn't that funny? I don't feel WOE. When I need to go somewhere, my car take me there. I've never had my electricity turned off (close maybe, but close only counts in horseshoes and hand grenades). My son has a strong, healthy body because he gets enough to eat; and people tell me I always look nice (regardless of hand-me-downs). I have dozens of pictures of my granddaughter and the eyes to see them with. When my son tells me "he doesn't know what he'd do without me in his life," when someone tells me "I'm glad you're my friend," when I'm on my knees and have the feelings of love, comfort, understanding and forgiveness flowing through me--these things fill my life with such joy and happiness that the WOES seem very unimportant.

My message is this. No matter what your problems or cares may be, have faith. My God gives me everything I need: joys and lessons. He knows all our needs. We're being given exactly what we need at any given point in time. We may not realize our need because we think mostly in terms of material needs. God works mostly on supplying our needs for spiritual growth, which lays the foundation for our daily acceptance to life, which brings true happiness. Our Higher Power gives us *"Serenity to accept the things we cannot change, courage to change what we can* (ourselves), *and wisdom to know the difference."*

19.   SLOW DOWN AND SMELL THE ROSES
(Gratitude)

Slow down and smell the roses on your busy, active day.
Slow down and breathe their fragrance, where they grow along life's way.

Take a minute of your lifetime to enjoy a pretty bloom.
Pluck a rose from nature's garden; it will brighten up your room.

Be not hasty in all your doings as you hurry through the day,
But enjoy ways God gives freely; smell the Roses while you may.

20.   SERENITY PRAYER
(Long version)

God, grant me
the serenity to accept the things I cannot change;
the courage to change the things I can;
the wisdom to know the difference.

Living one day at a time;
Enjoying one moment at a time;
Accepting hardship as the pathway to peace;

Taking, as He did, this sinful world as it is,
not as I would have it;
Trusting that He will make all things right
if I surrender to His Will;

That I may be reasonably happy in this life,
and supremely happy with Him forever in the next.
Amen.

21.   MY PROGRAM
(Having a direction)

Since I first came into the Fellowship, there
have been a lot of trials and tribulations, a lot of anger,
resentment and pain; a lot of confusion, fear, etc. But
without all these things, my awareness would not be at
the level it now is. Only through God have I been able
to come the distance I have today.

I wouldn't even have a program if it hadn't
been for God and the people I've come to know, love,
and appreciate in the program; the Fellowship, meetings, reading books; calling and talking with my sponsor and others who make up my support system. All

these things have helped me to put together a program of my own.

Without my Program, I'd still be floundering around somewhere out there, not having any direction, not having any discipline or guidance.

Today I have a place in life. I do belong. I have life, through the Program that God has given to me. And for that I am grateful today.

22.   GRATITUDE
(Not always easy)

Many times during the attendance of meetings, I hear the words grateful and gratitude. I have no doubt that when people say these words they mean them. For me having gratitude or being grateful is not always easy. For one thing, problems you don't have, you don't consider. Another is the tendency to take things for granted. And another is the habit of looking at what you don't have (materially) rather than being *grateful* for what you do have.

In order for me to be truly grateful, there are a few things that I must do. The first is to *stop*. The second is to become reflective, look at my past, and see where I am today. The third is to stay in the present and try to get materialism out of the picture. The fourth is to think of all the problems I could have and don't. The fifth, think of how much better I feel physically and mentally. Sixth, realize that my recovery is only a gift based on my spiritual growth from my Higher Power on a daily basis. Seventh, realize that in order to be truly grateful, I must gain more humility. I must know that I have to become more patient, tolerant, understanding and forgiving. Eighth, I must learn to turn it over, learn acceptance of myself and others, become more honest.

When I do all these things, *then* I can become grateful and have an attitude of gratitude.

23. A LETTER HOME
(Making amends)

Dear Mom & Dad:

I'm doing good. I didn't have to drink today. I didn't have to get high. I didn't eat the wrong foods today. I can't believe it. It's hard sometimes, but I just do what my friends tell me. I know it could be hard for you to understand all this 12-Step stuff, but I guess if you can just remember that it keeps me abstinent, there's no reason to complain about it. I know I was really awful to you guys, I mean you and Dad. I took money from you and stuff, and I was never really a daughter. I'm just doing what I'm told, and they say it really does get better. I don't really know about if you still love me or what, but I need these people right now. I need the Program. They keep talking about a Higher

Power, I mean like God. I guess I never really knew God would help me. I guess He is now because I'm not drunk or stoned and I didn't steal anything today. I sure did hurt you guys, didn't I? I really feel bad about stuff. I used to wish I was dead. But I'll make a deal with you, okay? I'll stay here and go to these meetings, stay straight and sober and try not to do awful stuff to people, and you guys can both sleep better tonite 'cause I been findin' out there really is a God.

Love,
Me

24. WHAT AN ORDER!
(A talk with my Higher Power)

What an order, I can't go through with it!
And a small, quiet voice said: *Be still and know that I am God.*

But God, you just don't understand, I am so alone and so very afraid.
Somewhere in my heart I heard: *I will not give you any more than you can handle.*

In my terror I screamed, I am not as capable as you think I am! Inside I am very small and very young. Oh God, I am so alone.

Again, a peaceful loving voice replied: *You have never been alone and you are not alone now. If you let me in, I will walk with you.*

I am too afraid, I cried; my heart hurts, and I just don't know what to do anymore. I put out my hand and no one was there. Oh God, I am so alone.

A gentle voice replied: *Putting out your hand is not enough. You must reach out with your whole being: your heart, soul, and mind. I will hold you in your fear and I will teach you past your youth.*

I am afraid, my God, that if I do this you will go away. I fall on my face and make so many mistakes. You may not love me if I let go completely.

A warmth and peace beyond my understanding filled my heart and mind. And I began to understand I didn't have to be alone if I didn't really want to be.

Very softly, very quietly, I heard: *The lesson isn't over until you've learned it completely. If you fail, if you fall, I will catch you. Ask for me and I will come. You only have to ask. You never have to be alone again. In times of great sorrow, I will send you comfort; when you are alone, I will send someone; in times of tremendous turmoil, I will grant you the gift of peace. Still, you must ask, even when you don't believe. And continue to reach out to your fellows, for they are as scared and alone*

*as you feel now. Life is difficult, but if you seek me and
follow what I say to your heart, then for any pain you live
through I will bless you with joy. For every time you
reach out in blind faith, I will grant you peace within
yourself and with your fellows.*

And I came to believe that a power greater
than myself, God, could and would restore me to
sanity. What I couldn't do for myself, God had. So I
reached out my heart, soul and mind to God. Thy will,
not mine, be done. Amen.

25.   GOD, I HATE MYSELF!

I'm on my knees this Wednesday night, hands
welded together in my struggle for the ultimate concentration, all stressed out, burned out and feeling like
a whipped puppy. I'm looking at the TV out of the
corner of my eye, trying not to focus on Oscar and Felix
doing the Odd Couple dance. My bed is still unmade
from last night, pillows strewn everywhere, sheets
crumpled, rumpled and dumped near the edge, cat
hair settling finally, offering a new dimension to the
elegance of Laura Ashley's Primrose and Melon cotton sheets. I hear sirens. I try to tune them out. I just
know the phone will ring. I wonder if I can pay my bills
this month. I wonder if I made my lunch. Yep, I did.
Unbelievable! I have to be at work early tomorrow!

Don't they get enough of my time? I am so frustrated. The wind whistles through the window frames. I hear conversation downstairs. I hear doors shut. I hear every noise in the entire universe.

I am in no mood for reverence. I am hardly the epitome of spiritual reception. Most of my brain cells are intimately plugged into the electrical socket of insanity. My heart, however, is in desperate need of my Lord.

Help me, Lord. This day stinks. I stink. I am full of self-loathing, self-pity, self-deprivation. I am full of self. I am sick to death of me. I am empty and cold and angry. I, I, I.

You are my child. I love all my children.

I can't help being this way. I am not capable of anything that's good. I make so many mistakes. I want to yell at people, snap at them, isolate myself from them, run away from home. I hate me!

Let go, my child. You are tired; you are sick; you are not bad.

I want to do good. I want to be what you want me to be. Help me, Lord. I can't do it alone. I have tried and tried; it seems never ending. How can I get better if I hate myself? I hate feeling this way!

Let go, my child. I have arms strong enough to hold you. There is no darkness from where I stand. Darkness and light are alike to me.

I can't. I feel scared. I feel like I will fall. I

don't think it's safe. There's too many people. There's too much pain. I want to feel better. I try and try but sometimes it feels like it's just too hard. It's just too much. I can't go on.

Do not question in the darkness what I give you in the light. Let go, my child. You are safe with me.

I am too scared! Don't you understand how frightening it is? You don't know what it's like to live in this head. You don't know how hard I try not to be afraid. It seems like I'm always afraid. I know it's stupid. I'm going out of my mind!

You come to me in pain. You tell me how you feel, and I hear you. You ask for my help, and I give it to you. Let go of the tears and the fears will lessen.

I'm sick of crying. That's all I ever do. I hate this! They say it gets better. I'm still a mess! How can you love me? I still don't sleep well! I still hide from people! I still can't call when I want to! Is that the way you want me to be?

I want you to be happy.

Then help me!

You have it. I am here for you always, to the end. I will give you what you need. Let go, my child, and know that I am God.

Oh, please, God, keep me safe. I turn my life and my will over to your care. I believe that you care. I am hanging off the edge of a cliff, clinging so tightly to a thin, spineless branch, wriggling and fighting for my life, thinking the stupid twig will keep me safe from falling. I hold on to what I know. It's hard to believe in what I haven't seen. I still think I know best. I still don't trust you. God, I hate myself! Help me, Lord. This branch isn't strong enough to keep me from falling!

Let it go.

Oh God, if I let go, I'll fall! I'll die! Don't ask me to let go of this branch. It's all I have to hold on to!

Let go and you will find safety and comfort.

Let go and I will find safety and comfort. Right. I'll slip through the sky and land in the pits of hell again. Will you catch me?

I will be waiting.

Will you catch me?

I will be there.

If I let go, I mean *if* I let go, will you promise to stay with me until I feel better?

I am with you always.

God, I bet (sniffle) ... I just bet (sniffle) ... you know what would be nice? If I let go, maybe I'll fall, just maybe, I'll fall right into your arms. Oh God, help me!

Let go, my child, and I will give you rest.

The night noise still rattles the walls; the expressways and trains still plead for my attention; TV wails with nonsense; and the Primrose and Melon cotton sheets still wind up in a lump. I have cried and sniffled and the kleenex is gone. My eyes have puffed up and my nose has ceased to function. But I feel loved. *I feel loved!* Maybe tomorrow will be crazy; maybe I'll forget. But just maybe, God and I ... well, maybe we really talked.

26.   JUDGING OTHERS

Does this sound familiar? You hear about someone's behavior or character defects from some-one else. Then you observe this person (based on your opinion ASSUMING what you were told is true) exhibiting this kind of behavior, and of course this is proof enough for you. So naturally you cannot contain your resentment, jealousy, fear, etc., and you feel you must share this in turn with another person instead of your sponsor.

Perhaps, if you're lucky, the things that you say will be kept in confidence by this other person; but as the saying goes, "As soon as you ask someone 'please don't say anything,' you've given them the reason to say it."

But as most often happens, eventually the original party with this character defect will get wind of what's being said. God knows how sensitive we in recovery are!! Who knows what this person will decide to do? Maybe they won't go to "that" meeting any more. Maybe friendships will be destroyed. Maybe they will drop out of the Fellowship altogether.

If your conscience starts working on you, maybe, just maybe, you may start wondering if what has been said isn't true. Maybe this person doesn't have this character defect. Maybe you'll wonder if you really know this person and understand their motives. You might start asking yourself questions like: "Have I ever done the same thing myself?" "Maybe I was just assuming because of what it LOOKED LIKE." "Don't I have character defects too?" "Have I ever talked with this person and tried to understand?" "Do I really have the right to judge what's in another person's heart, especially when I've been the brunt of another's gossip and, understanding my own motives, knew full well it wasn't true?"

As Shakespeare once said, "What's done cannot be undone." We must eventually pay the consequences for our actions. But we do have a solution, through the 12 Steps, that can, if an honest effort and willingness on our part is made, set right these wrongs.

We can work a 4th, 5th, or 10th Step to enable us to see what character defect of OUR OWN (anger, fear, jealousy) was responsible for OUR ACTION. We can work the 6th and 7th Step if WE honestly don't want to keep behaving this way. We can work the 10th Step and admit WE were wrong in OUR ACTION even if our opinion of this person remains the same.

And most importantly, discuss with our spon-

sors FIRST how to make the amends and what should
be said. If we do this on our own, we may be clearing
our own conscience at another's expense and so fulfill
the warning *except when to do so would injure them or
others.*

27. ARE YOU AN ACTIVE MEMBER?

Are you an active member
The kind that would be missed
Or are you just contented
That your name is on the list?
Do you attend the meetings
And mingle with the flock
Or do you stay at home
And just criticize and knock?
Do you take an active part
To help the work along
Or are you just satisfied
To be the kind that "Just Belongs"?
Do you ever visit a member
Who is bedridden or sick
Or leave the work to just a few
And talk about the "Clique"?
There's quite a program scheduled
And we'll appreciate if you, too,
Will come and help us out!
So come to the meetings more often

And help out with hand and heart.
Don't be just another member
But take an active part.
Think it over, my sisters,
You know right from wrong,
Are you an active member
Or do you just belong?

28.   A WINNER IS . . .

SOMEONE WHO loses, and comes back to fight again.
SOMEONE WHO makes mistakes, and admits them, and apologizes sincerely.
SOMEONE WHO accepts themselves, but without complacency.
SOMEONE WHO accepts others' rights to be as they are, without criticism.
SOMEONE WHO asks "How are you?" and really wants to know.
SOMEONE WHO listens, and hears.
SOMEONE WHO sees without blinders or rose-colored glasses.
SOMEONE WHO is honest.
SOMEONE WHO strives to be the best that they can be, and hopes it makes a difference that they lived at all, because we've all been given a second chance.

SOMEONE WHO believes that success in the Program and the credit for it belongs not to themselves but to a higher power.

SOMEONE WHO can ask for help.

SOMEONE WHO's not looking for an idol, but recognizes the good in each member, thereby being disappointed by none.

SOMEONE WHO is brand new, *and* hurting, *and* keeps coming back.

SOMEONE WHO works *all* of the 12 Steps, and practices these principles in *all* their affairs.

SOMEONE WHO is humble.

29.   CHANGE
(Irritating but necessary)

For the first three years of my recovery, my partner made it possible for me to attend any evening meetings I wished to. He realized, very soon after I accepted my addiction, that I desperately needed meetings as insurance. However, I didn't need meetings chosen at random; I needed the safety and comfort of regular meetings at my home group where I felt I really belonged.

Now my partner has evening commitments which make it much more difficult for me to attend my home group meetings, which are all held at night. He was available to stay home with the children for a long time, and now it is my turn to tailor my schedule to suit his. This is not only an opportunity for me to make amends to him for the past, but also an opportunity for me to change and therefore grow. A comment I've heard in the Program, "You're not required to like it; you're only required to *do* it!" is what I need to remember in times of change, when I need the faith to break away from the familiar and rechart my course into the future.

Times of change draw on every reserve I have: faith, hope, love, inspiration and anything else I'm able to absorb from the Program; and I'm well aware that, without these spiritual reserves of strength, I wouldn't be able to face many of the changes and adjustments I have already handled successfully in recovery.

My writing today began with a pang of guilt that I wasn't repaying that debt of spiritual strength to the group that has helped me grow from a child into a responsible adult. However, writing and sharing my thoughts with you has dispelled that guilt and has reminded me that I am not alone. There are members all over the world who have feelings, emotions and attitudes similar to mine. And when I look at myself in a noncritical way, I realize that I'm doing the very best, just for today, that I'm capable of doing at this point in my recovery.

30.   ON BEING YOUNG AND FEMALE IN ALCOHOLICS ANONYMOUS
(Overcoming obstacles)

"Was totally defeated by alcohol, as it was the pain of my alcoholism that forced me to reach out for help through Alcoholics Anonymous."

I am an alcoholic - a person who is powerless over alcohol. I am also young and a female. Two of the past three Communications Meetings have been of particular relevance to "the role of women in A.A." and "the role of young people in A.A." The fact that these two meetings were called suggests that the rapidly growing membership of both women and young people is causing some concern. Are we ready and strong enough in our own individual and collective sobrieties to be able to carry the message of recovery to those two groups of sufferers? These questions have arisen because the Fellowship in the past and still today is predominantly male with the vast majority of members being over thirty.

I came to the Fellowship three years ago at the age of twenty. I was totally defeated by alcohol, as it was the pain of my alcoholism that forced me to reach out for help through Alcoholics Anonymous. Many well-meaning members who were pleased to see one so young, told me that it was good that I arrived here before I suffered the years of pain which they had gone through. I reacted, and felt that my own pain for which I had come had been belittled.

Thus I hit my first barrier to feeling secure within the Fellowship. That initial sense of belonging started to be undermined as I was identified by others as a "Baby Alky" who had not really felt the tortures of alcoholism.

Next came the problems of identity and, coinciding with that, dependency. All my life I had been known as Geoff and Mary's daughter. Very rarely had I been given my own identity as Chris. I had come to this Fellowship a totally dependent person. I was not only dependent on alcohol but also on other people for my own sense of security, identity, sense of self-worth, etc. I no longer found these in alcohol, parents, material things or friends. I was very open to latching onto others to fill this particular need.

Around the Fellowship, I found, and they found me, many members willing to play mother and father to me. Once again I reacted, as this was dependency I had been fighting for years, and yet I could not get out of it. As well as this, I felt that I was not being treated as an equal, as a fellow alcoholic. Fortunately, I had not married and been identified as so and so's wife. Again it was suggested that perhaps I should pretty myself up and go out and find a man; I would make some fellow a lovely wife. As a woman, it seemed I had to find my identity through a man.

It was also presumed that as I became well, I would start to wear makeup, dress like a lady, marry and have children. These attitudes were expressed to me directly at meetings of A.A. My lifestyle today does not fit this bill, and it has only been through the Program of A.A. that I have been given the courage to be me, Chris.

Further problems arose with identification as an alcoholic, and my own identifying at meetings. It was suggested that I look for the similarities and not the differences. I did identify as a practicing alcoholic, but I found it extremely hard to gauge just what I had lost through my drinking. In reality, I never lost anything because I never had anything in the first place to lose: no monetary gains, no self-respect, no identity, no family, no friends, no anything! Alcohol had just brought me to my knees much quicker. And so, when I did stop drinking, I didn't have anything to regain.

I could not say that I had "got" anything or anyone back. I could not see or feel the immediate benefits of sobriety. However, a few things did leave me, e.g., my thieving and prostitution for alcohol, hangovers and blackouts. But my life did not change to any great degree as a result of my simply putting down the drink. At meetings I heard the few vague references to sexuality usually in the form of men who were having affairs with numerous "chicks," wife bashing, dirty jokes and happy marriages today.

It is quite acceptable for a male to deviate from the straight and narrow, excepting of course that of homosexuality, but it is still not so for the woman. How could I ever express my own past experiences with both men and women to any one person, let alone from the floor of an A.A. meeting? And this definitely held me back in my sobriety as my guilt feelings of my past just grew and blew right out of proportion.

Still I very rarely heard a woman speak of how she was degraded even more sexually through her alcoholism, of rape, prostitution, seeking security through men, fears, anxieties, etc. Why? Because she was afraid of ridicule, of rejection, of becoming the prey of "sick" men, and was told straight out that we were only here for our alcoholism. Yet men could still talk of their ill treatment of women and on many occasions get the laughs.

I had the same problem as a young person, when identifying at meetings. The Big Book tells me to share what I was like, what happened, and what I'm like now. I attempted to do this and so I often spoke about my own emotional state, the way I related to people, sexuality, and the various aspects of me which contributed to my practicing alcoholism, my state of mind, and consequently, my sobriety today.

I was told not to analyze myself, that I should only speak of my drinking and how I got to A.A. I did this when I first came around the Fellowship. I conformed and told you what I drank, how I drank, who I drank with and where, my physical and financial condition, how I got to A.A., and that things would get better so long as I kept coming to meetings. Within fourteen months I was drunk again. I had not disclosed anything of myself to anyone. I was still carrying the same load of guilt and more, fears, anxieties, hangups, loneliness, resentments, etc., with which I had come into A.A.

I did not feel a sense of belonging in A.A. even though I knew my answer was here. I was full of fear of drinking again, of being found out and rejected for having problems other than alcoholism; e.g., my fear of being autistic, my not being attracted to men.

I had not been given an alternative way of life, nor had anyone shared with me the tools for finding that alternative which is the Twelve Steps of Alcoholics Anonymous.

But fortunately I kept coming to meetings, and finally a member shared with me, as fellow alcoholics, his own experience of recovery through the Twelve Steps. It was from here that I once again revived hope and saw that truly there was a lot more to my disease than simply alcohol; and that in order to be freed from myself, I needed to do more than simply avoid picking up the first drink and going to plenty of A.A. meetings. I needed to put those Twelve Steps, which hang on banners behind the chairperson, into my life until they became an integral part of it. And I needed to start right now by putting a conscious effort into them.

Through utter desperation I was able to do this and I immediately started to feel the promises of the Program. I learned about sobriety and how to attain and maintain it from the first 164 pages of the Big Book which decorates the table at meetings. I also learned how to apply these things to my life through the sharing of experience with the Twelve Steps of Recovery at my home group. Here I found in-depth sharing of the person, and I was able truly to identify and gain the support and encouragement I so desperately needed. There are now Step Groups opened in other areas.

It is only through the Twelve Steps that I have been able to find and feel the strength of my Higher Power which is today my defense against the first drink. I am able to share this and build upon this strength today through the practice of the Program and via meetings. I have found myself and others today, and consequently my life is taking on a new direction and is growing, as is my sobriety. I love the Fellowship of A.A. as I love the Program and my Higher Power. My bond with the Fellowship is our common stepping stones to living, the Program of recovery. I need a peer group with whom to grow, and I find that peer group with Alcoholics Anonymous.

31.   COMING TO RELY UPON "THAT GOD THING" *(Step 3)*

". . . TO THE CARE of God as I understand him."

There was a time when reading or hearing that, I arrogantly would have said to myself, "Oh, no, there's some more of that God thing again. Why don't they give it a rest?"

So, if you're like I used to be, go ahead and turn the page, because this is going to be about God.

After I began to realize (believe it or not) that I *needed* this God thing, I wasn't real sure how to go about a "God of my own understanding." Realizing that my best thinking is what got me here, I decided to seek some help in this matter. I bought books about spirituality, talked to other members, and as they said, I tried to take what I could use and leave the rest. I wrote down everything I thought God was and exactly what I expected God to do for me. (At the time, it never occurred to me that God might have a few expectations of me.)

As I began to experience spirituality through attendance at meetings, time with my sponsor, and prayer, my belief in a Higher Power began to change, mature, and grow stronger. Eventually, this spiritual belief turned into a means by which to live and interact with God, myself and others.

Step Three reads: "We made a decision to turn our will and our lives over to the care of God *as we understood Him.*" What I'd like to express is how I perceive the "care of God." *Webster's Dictionary* defines *care* as: (1) An object or source of worry; (2) Protection; supervision; charge; (3) To be concerned or interested; (4) To have a liking or attachment; (5) Caution in avoiding harm or danger; heedfulness.

Translated in terms of my relationship with God, I believe that when I turn my will over, God worries about *me* and takes the process of worrying from me. This allows me to experience serenity and peace of mind: no more rats pacing on the treadmill.

When I turn my life over, I experience God's protection and supervision. I am in my Higher Power's charge (not, *I* am in charge). God is concerned and interested in what is spiritually, emotionally and physically best for me (such as the removal of my desire for my addictions). As in any good relationship, a loving God feels a liking or attachment to me.

Even in recovery, there are many times when I'm not aware of behaviors, actions, attitudes, or expressions that are harmful to me and to others, so God helps me to be cautious, to avoid doing harm or getting in danger (God's grace). God places obstacles or

people in my path to make me aware of the will which
isn't mine.

32.   THE CHILD WITHIN

Little girl inside of me
I'm surprised that you're still there
Patiently waiting for me to see
How much you need my care

Little girl, your tears are felt
They fall upon my own face
And all that pain that you've been dealt
I wish I could erase

Little girl, I'll understand
If you can't trust me just now
But it's possible I've found a plan
To work this out somehow

Little girl, I'm going to hear
All the things you need from me
And from now on I'll hold you near
With love eternally

Little girl, your fear I feel
I wish I could make it subside

But that's the price for being real
And I'm just as scared inside

Little girl, a world's out there
Let's go see it together
Let's think of things that we can share
And pray it lasts forever.

33.   BEING INVOLVED
   *(Attending meetings and helping
   newcomers)*

Early in recovery, I was told that the best
definition for love is action. When you love someone,
you do things for that person for the simple joy of doing
it -- no strings attached.

I was also told that I should go to every
meeting with only one thought in mind: What can I
add to this meeting by being here? With this attitude,
I have never attended a bad meeting, nor have I ever
attended one meeting too many.

I was told when I took Step Three that self-
concern had no more place in my life, that I was God's
problem now. With Step Seven, I was reminded that
God is the doer, and that the best way to get myself off
my own mind, so that God could do His work, was to

get involved with helping newcomers. I have been
actively involved for more than eight years now, and it
works! I plan to stay involved, too. Why change a
winning formula?

34.   SIMPLE QUESTIONS
(*Minding my own business*)

One of the first things I heard after getting
into the Program was that I must learn to deal with only
those problems which are mine.

To me, this was a polite way of saying, "Mind
my own business." Since it has always been my nature
to feel that I know what is best for everyone, deciding
what is my business and what is *not* has been extremely
difficult.

Although we are provided with numerous
slogans as tools, I could not find one which quite
seemed to fit for this glaring defect of mine.

I decided that perhaps I could devise some
personal tools of my own which would help. I came up
with two questions which force me to look honestly at
myself when I feel the urge to give unsolicited advice or
to otherwise become involved in things which do not
concern me:

            (1)   Is that your problem?
            (2)   Did anyone ask your opinion?

It's amazing how frequently the answer to both of these questions is NO!

This keeps my Program simple and helps keep me comfortable in recovery.

35. MY EMOTIONS ARE MY TEACHERS

I read somewhere that it is normal to feel anger, frustration, resentment, depression, joy and love. Some are negative; some are positive. I asked my sponsor about "emotions," and she said my emotions are my teachers.

"How can that be?" I asked. "My emotions usually get me into trouble." She explained that emotions are not bad; they are normal. And they can be very helpful if I will just learn from them. "But how do I learn from them?" was my next question. My sponsor went on to say that when I am feeling some emotion such as anger or resentment, I need to stop and do a quick Fourth Step (or Tenth Step). She said I should ask myself *who* is causing me to feel angry, *what* are they doing to upset me, and *why* am I letting them upset me. Am I afraid; am I jealous; am I guilty? What's "bugging" me?

Then she said to consider what I can do to get rid of the anger. She said that action is the magic word, action to work the Steps, especially Steps Four and

Twelve. By focusing my attention on helping someone else, I get the spotlight off of *me*. I can go to one of our clubs or groups and seek out a newcomer.

As a last resort, I can take out my Twelve Step list or my group member list and call a few people just to say "hello and have a good day"!

Yes, my emotions are my teachers. They teach me to stop being so self-centered, to change my focus to others, to change my activities from seething inside to helping others outside.

My sponsor was right. ACTION is the Magic Word!

36.   GETTING BETTER

Gratitude is foremost on my mind these days. Before the Program I was filled with hopelessness, fear and hate. Most of all I hated myself. It's not like that today. My life is better than it has ever been. Recovery has not always been easy, but it has *always* been better than my active addiction days. God has been good to me. He has given me the courage to look at myself and helped me to make changes. With God's help, my relationship with my husband is better, though there was a time in early recovery when I thought our marriage was over. I am also back in a profession I love. I still have a lot of work to do on myself; but, if I don't use, go to meetings, read the Big Book and work the

Program, I will get better. I am very grateful for the
Program.

37. AN OPEN LETTER TO SPONSEES

Since you are very important to me, I hope
you will keep this to refer to at times, especially when
there may be uncertainties and you cannot reach me
for a personal explanation or reminder.

When I agreed to sponsor you, it was to help
us both maintain what has to be first in our lives:
abstinence. I would learn from you, and I have learned
from you, and I thank you. You have grown in the
Program, and that you can also take thanks for; you accepted and took advantage of what we had to offer. I
have helped carry it to you, but I did not give it. Neither
will I take the blame if you choose to forget what you
have learned.

At first, I was very ready to verbalize my
opinions on many topics because, in the early stages of
recovery, a new member is much like a child who needs
guidance. Maybe I offered suggestions in areas other
than "*do not use and go to meetings*." Now there are
times when you ask an opinion on other issues and I do
not give it. That is because I feel you are ready now to
think for yourself, and in order to grow you must do
this.

However, on questions about recovery I will still be ready to give you what I consider to be my best answer.

Do not ask or expect me to solve your day-to-day problems. I am only human, but you and God have an arrangement that will best fit. God has promised you'll not be given more than your brain and resources can handle. I cannot cheat you out of your right to grow by interfering with that. If, being human, I should try, please don't let me. I might make that mistake because I care about you, but remind me that all we agreed upon was that I would do whatever I could to help you recover.

The exception is if I think you may be doing something that will endanger your recovery. Then I will become very much a sponsor. *And vocal!!!*

You have always been a special person to me because of what we have shared. If you feel any time someone else could help you more and would like to change sponsors, I not only approve, I *insist* upon it. Working the Program is our priority, and whatever we have to do to attain this goal is what must be done. You would still be special and I would look forward to seeing you at meetings. If you should feel the need to avoid me because of *"guilt,"* then I have not been a very good example for you and did not pass on that *people*, *places*, and *things* cannot take precedence over recovery.

Whether or not I remain your sponsor has no bearing on the fact that I want us always to be friends. GOD BLESS YOU.

38.   FORGIVENESS

To forgive a person in any circumstances costs us nothing. Say that they have defrauded me, injured my reputation, attempted my life; and suppose such an enemy is in my power, what does it cost me to forgive them? Let us see: To reduce them to poverty would make me no richer; to destroy their peace would not restore my own; to hurt them would not heal me; or to cast a blot on their reputation would restore no luster to my name; to take their life would not insure me against the stroke of death, nor lengthen my life by a single hour.

It is a happy memory that remembers kindness and forgets offenses. It is far more noble to conquer one's passion than to crush a foe; and sweeter than gratified revenge are their feelings who, when their enemy hungers, feed them; when they thirst, gives them water. In so doing, people exhibit somewhat of the nature, and taste something of the happiness of God.

39.   SUCCESS

Success is speaking words of praise
In cheering other people's ways.
In doing just the best you can
With every task and every plan.
It's silence when your speech would hurt,
Politeness when your neighbor's curt.
It's deafness when the scandal flows,
And sympathy with others' woes.
It's loyalty when duty calls.
It's courage when disaster falls.
It's patience when the hours are long.
It's found in laughter and in song.
It's in the silent time of prayer,
In happiness and in despair,
In all of life and nothing less,
We find the thing we call success.

40.   THE DRIVER'S SEAT

So many times we in 12-Step Programs hear
the remark, "Get out of the driver's seat and turn our
will and our lives over to the care of God, as we
understand Him," which is the Third Step of our Program. What do we turn over? Do we sit back and let
Him take care of us twenty-four hours of each day? In

a way, this would be nice for some people if it were possible. We would become a machine with God just pushing the buttons.

The majority of everyday trials and tribulations we can handle with the free will God gave us. For a number of years, I could handle my addiction with the will He gave me, without too much trouble. Then came the day when I could no longer handle it, and then the trouble came. The reason for the trouble was that I didn't have the humility to slide over and say, "God, take over, because I can't drive safely anymore." I spent years fighting humility and had nothing but trouble with my addiction.

Our addiction is not the only thing for which we must get out of the driver's seat. Anger, envy, jealousy, hate are among the character defects that must be removed. I'm still an addict, just as I still have all of those traits, and each one, when I stay in the driver's seat, can cause me trouble to the point of mental collapse.

When any character defect has gone overboard, we must slide out of the driver's seat. It takes humility and prayer to get God to take over. It's not like driving a car; you don't stop and say to Him, "take over." God may be sitting right alongside you, but He won't take over unless you have the true humility to let Him.

Serenity is knowing yourself, and praying each

day for help in correcting the character defects you don't have the ability to control yourself. Only you and God know the defects of character that you can't handle alone.

Join hands with Him. It's a great life if you do.

41. THE HEART OF THE PROGRAM
(Step 2)

The most interesting characteristic of the Second Step is its effect on new persons in the Program. Some newcomers, perhaps most, already have accepted the doctrine that there is a Power greater than themselves. For others more cynical, they have difficulty believing that there is *anything* real unless it is another person or thing.

Up to this point, the newcomers may have liked what they heard during meetings. The 24-hour-a-day plan for living, the Fellowship and the familiarity of the language talked, the idea of helping others, all of these appeal to them as logical, pleasant and practical. But now comes "this God stuff." The atheist or agnostic might think it's enough to make the blood in their veins turn to acid.

Yet the Second Step, in my opinion, is the very heart of the Program. Without it, the most carefully planned approach to recovery fails; without it, the most stubborn and determined fall. Unless there is acceptance of a Power greater than ourselves, the other Steps become meaningless.

The words "came to believe" suggest a wise and gradual approach. One of our slogans can be applied: "Easy does it."

When we accept the fact that there is a Power greater than ourselves, it is not too difficult to call on this Power for the courage and wisdom necessary to face even a bleak reality. In other words, we have found an understanding and helpful friend who cannot fail us. We are no longer alone!

Even the most cynical of our fellows would surely admit that the sun rises, that the stars are in the sky even though they can't be seen through the clouds. So they do have faith in *some* things. If you're having trouble with Step 2, look around you. There are millions of people in this world in recovery. Many of them, too, had trouble with the Second Step. But they continued to *try to believe* and they *kept an open mind*! Today they are well. If they remain "in" the Program, they will stay well.

42.   DEAR GOD

Dear God,
I have no idea where I am going.
I do not see the road ahead of me.
I cannot know for certain where it will end.

Nor do I really know myself, and the fact that I am actually doing so.

But I believe this.

I believe that the desire to please You does in fact please You.

I hope I have that desire in everything I do.

I hope I never do anything apart from that desire.

And I know that if I do this, You will lead me by the right road though I may know nothing about it at the time.

Therefore, I will trust you always, for though I may seem to be lost and in the shadow of death, I will not be afraid because I know you will never leave me to face my troubles alone.

43.   CHANGING ATTITUDES ON CHANGE

There are only two things I am sure of about change: (1) it's consistent, and (2) I don't like it. All my life I've hung onto people, places and things long past the time to let them go.

Recently it was brought home to me when I moved into a new apartment. I bitched and moaned about the place I lived in for ten years, but it was familiar; it was home.

There is no comparison between the apartment I have now and the one I just left. After twenty-five years, I again have a dishwasher and garbage disposal. I have room. I have storage space. The area is attractive. I wouldn't need to apologize if people came to visit.

Yet, for days, I had that lonely, lost feeling of a person displaced. I no longer had a home, a haven, a place I could be comfortable. I didn't want to come here at night, but I didn't have any place else to go. I would sit here and ask myself, "Who am I trying to impress? Who do I think I am? I don't need all this." What I was really saying is, "I don't deserve to live in a nice place. *It is not familiar to me.* I belong where I was. *I don't like change.*"

I can remember years ago owning a little foreign car that I hated. Yet when I left that car as a trade-in, I almost cried. And every time I saw that car afterwards, I still thought of it as mine.

I can remember feeling so lonely and so alone that I would start thinking of all my boyfriends, and even old husbands, and thinking life with them had not been that bad. Again, wanting what I knew.

Once I even wrote to my first husband years after I had divorced my second one. Thank God I never got a response.

I realize today (sometimes after several days or weeks of agony) that it isn't so much that I don't like change--I fear it! To accept change I have to change my thinking, my attitudes and my actions, and that to me is "scary." My mind says it is much easier to stay with the familiar, whether it be good or bad.

This Program is slowly teaching me that it is not change that makes life so difficult for me but my resistance to it.

My problem today is that just as soon as I accept the change, it changes again!

44. LIFE IS A CELEBRATION

Mend a quarrel.
Seek out a forgotten friend.
Dismiss suspicion and replace it with trust.
Write a friendly letter. Share a treasure.
Give a soft answer. Encourage another.
Manifest your loyalty in word and deed.
Keep a promise. Find the time.
Forego a grudge.
Forgive an enemy. Listen . . .
Acknowledge any wrongdoing.
Try to understand.
Examine your demands on others.
Think of someone else first.
Be kind. Be gentle. Laugh a little.
Smile more. Be happy. Show your gratitude.
Welcome a stranger.
Speak your love. Speak it again.
Live it again.
Life is a celebration!

45. THE SERENITY PRAYER
(An interpretation)

GOD GRANT ME THE SERENITY . . . I have
known peace, the peace that comes in front of a fire-
place on a cozy winter's night, the peace of the mountains; but when I would leave the mountains, the peace
would leave me. When the fire went out or the phone
rang, the peace would be gone. Peace came rarely and
went quickly, a mood conjured by myself for myself.
Serenity is different. It is all that peace is, but it stays.
It carries over. It is with me and in me. Nothing
disturbs it. It is given; therefore, it cannot be taken
away.

TO ACCEPT THE THINGS I CANNOT CHANGE
. . . One accepts when one receives. To understand, to
take into the mind without debate as one receives a
gift, this is acceptance. Serenity precedes acceptance.
It must. There is order to this. My mind must be calm
in order to understand what you are saying. To listen
to you without debate, I must not be afraid of you.
With the gift of serenity, I am able to accept people and
circumstances as they are, not as I want them to be or
as I think they should be. I am willing to accept the bad
as well as the good, because it is all a part of the plan.
When I accept a situation as it is, when I accept you just
as you are, I have stopped playing God.

COURAGE TO CHANGE THE THINGS I CAN
. . . When my ego is involved and there's a calculated risk, I'm going to be gutsy, not courageous. It takes guts to ski a steep trail; I alone will be rewarded. Courage is different. There is always a parenthesis of fear in courage; the risk becomes minor. This parenthesis remains a void of fear until it is filled by God. There is no ego in a courageous act. Courage can ask for help. It is often something done for someone else, or it may be something I am not attracted to doing at all. I may lose by doing it. The courageous act is often the unpopular choice, to do or not to do. The results are seldom only mine. It requires more of me than I want to think I can do, alone. After it is finished, gratitude to someone or something is usually in order. Courage requires a moral strength not of myself. This strength is given by faith.

AND WISDOM TO KNOW THE DIFFERENCE
. . . Wisdom is God's own conversation with me. Often He speaks through books or other people. Wisdom can be found merely by listening to others after I develop the ability to hear it in their words. To recognize wisdom, I must have compassion for others, which gives me insight rather than knowledge of myself. Facing reality encourages recognition of wisdom, because wisdom is always truth.

46.   I PRAY FOR CALMNESS
(Step 11)

I will try to keep my life calm and unruffled. This is my great task, to find peace and acquire serenity. I must not harbor disturbing thoughts. No matter what fears, worries and resentments I may have, I must try to think of constructive things, until calmness comes.

I will come to God in faith and God will give me a new way of life. This new way of life will alter my whole existence, the words I speak, the influence I have. They will spring from the life within me. I see how important is the work of a person that has this new way of life. The words and the example of such a person can have a wide influence for good in the world.

I will learn to overcome myself, because every blow to selfishness is used to shape the real, eternal, unperishable me. As I overcome myself, I gain the power which God releases in my soul. And I too will be victorious. It is not the difficulties of life that I have to conquer, so much as my own selfishness.

I will relax and not get tense. I will have no fear, because everything will work out in the end. I will learn soul-balance and poise in a vacillating, changing world. I will claim God's power and use it because if I do not use it, it will be withdrawn. As long as I get back to God and replenish my strength after each task, no work can be too much.

I believe that God had already seen my heart's needs before I was conscious of those needs myself. I believe that God was already preparing the answer. God does not have to be petitioned with sighs and tears and much speaking. God has already anticipated my every want and need. I will try to see this, as my Higher Power's plans unfold in my life.

I will never forget to say thank you to God, even on grayest days. My attitude will be one of humility and gratitude. Saying thank you to God is a daily practice that is absolutely necessary. If a day is not one of thankfulness, the practice has to be repeated until it becomes so. Gratitude is a necessity for those who seek to live a better life.

In these times of quiet meditation, try more and more to set your hopes on the grace of God. Know that whatever the future may hold, it will hold more and more of good. Do not set all your hopes and desires on material things; there is weariness in an abundance of things. Set your hopes on spiritual things so that you may grow spiritually. Learn to rely on God's power more and more, and in that reliance you will have an insight into the greater value of the things of the spirit.

You were meant to be at home and comfortable in the world. Yet some people live a life of quiet desperation. This is the opposite of being at home and at peace in the world. Let your peace of mind be evident to those around you. Let others see that you are comfortable, and seeing it, know that it springs from your trust in a Higher Power. Faith takes the sting out of the winds of adversity and brings peace even in the midst of struggle.

I pray that I may be calm and let nothing upset me. I pray that I may not let material things control me and choke out spiritual things.

47. GETTING IN TOUCH WITH OURSELVES

Change is difficult for all of us. The older we get, the more difficult it becomes. We all want to be able to predict what is going to happen in order to prepare our defenses and control situations. We don't like surprises. We fear the unknown.

We want things definite and certain. We don't like our expectancies frustrated, our habits disturbed, or our stereotypes challenged.

Habits are helpful. They are our way through life. It would be most burdensome if we had to stop and consider each time we wanted to type a page or drive a car.

But when it comes to interpersonal relations, values, new ideas, growth, the challenges of a changing society, some habits can be a handicap. They can lead us to believe we should not make moves, not ask questions, not look deeper, leave it to others who "know better."

The result can be that we conform to other people's statements about life and reality; become less responsive to ourselves, our own feelings and convictions; to what we truly feel, believe and want.

Sometimes we hide or even repress our true feelings because we are afraid to acknowledge that we believe something unusual or different or because they might require us to face something we would prefer not to face. Thus we can become dishonest and less real and program ourselves never to look into our deeper consciousness.

When we ignore our feelings, we cut ourselves off from experience and from reality, because experience is the best way of coming to know reality.

Getting in touch with ourselves, our experience, is a prerequisite of really knowing the God of our understanding and other people.

In our society, with all its business and distractions, privacy, intimacy, reflection, and quiet require planning and effort.

Ask yourself, "Is it at all possible, beginning now, that I could do the things I like more frequently or for longer periods and the things I dislike less frequently and for shorter periods?" What would be the consequences if I did the things I like to do more often? What would be the consequences if I did less often the things I do not like to do?

Too many people are waiting for some distant day (which never comes) when they will be able to do the things they want. There is truth in the saying, "Live now! Grasp the day and the moment."

What can you do to grasp the moment and change your way of life, even in a very small way?

48. CHARACTER DEFECTS
(Steps 6 and 7)

When I first came to the Program, I wanted all the good things people had, but I didn't want to work for them. Oh, I worked the Steps -- at least the ones I thought I needed. And when it came to Steps 6 and 7, I was ready and willing to have God remove my shortcomings -- should I have any, of course. I had no idea what they were because I didn't think I needed Steps 4 and 5. But I prayed, vaguely, that should God see any shortcomings, I was ready for my Higher Power to remove them. Of humility, the principle of Step 7, I had none.

As I progressed in the Program of recovery, I was made aware of many character defects and of just how blind I had been to them. Mercifully, God showed me only what I was ready to see.

I became depressed and thought I could never

be forgiven for or relieved from these shortcomings. This depression, I discovered, was not humility, but another form of "playing God," believing my character defects more powerful than God's forgiveness.

Then, when I recognized Who had the power and who was powerless, I had to decide if I was "entirely ready" to ask God to remove my shortcomings. After all, my character defects were what made up my personality, and I was pretty much in love with who I was. Self will had been my god for a lifetime. I was afraid, not knowing that something better would take the place of my character defects.

With all the honesty I was capable of at the time, I worked the Steps in order, one through 6, then 7, asking as humbly as I could that God remove my shortcomings. They did not disappear. I was not struck pure.

Then I was made aware that character defects are like addiction. I couldn't keep using and expect God to relieve my addiction. Neither could I keep practicing my character defects and expect God to remove them.

I was going to have to develop a new set of habits, to work against myself; and as I practiced these new habits, the old habits/character defects would begin to die.

And so began the living part of the Program: the daily striving to change, to let go and receive more.

It doesn't happen overnight. It takes years of practice.
I have not yet been struck pure. I am not a saint. But
I claim, accept and am grateful for spiritual progress.

49.   GETTING HONEST

How important is honesty to our Program of
recovery? In "How It Works" it says that *"Rarely have
we seen a person fail . . . those who do not recover . . .
(are) usually men and women who are constitutionally
incapable of being honest with themselves."* And that is
the only requirement for failure to stay abstinent
mentioned there. It doesn't say that this Program
won't work if we are unemployed, without a relationship or in poor health. It says only that we need to be
honest with ourselves, God, and another human being.

What is meant by honesty in the Program?
Some ideas we've heard are: "getting into agreement
with the facts," "to thine own self be true," and
"absence of theft." When honesty is first mentioned,
most of our minds gravitate to the idea of theft. After
all, a lot of us have never heard it applied in any other
way before! And so when we think of theft we think of
material things, all the way from taking paper clips
home from work to armed robbery. The value of what
we took really mattered little; it's how the act of
stealing made us feel that drove us to using to kill the

emotional pain of letting family, friends and God down by being a thief.

But as we listen, we find that there is more to this concept of honesty than stealing material things! We hear that we have to get honest about our part in all situations causing us emotional pain. We have to get into agreement with the facts of our lives, examine our motives, and eliminate self-deception. It is suggested that we do this with another human being. We have been talking to ourselves for years and kept coming up with the same answers (ones that enabled us to use); however, an outside listener can often lend great enlightenment, if we let them.

This, we say, is painful; why go through it? We become honest because it is the truth that sets us free. We have found that if we illuminate every area of our lives with truth, we begin to be set free from a painful past. Our egos are punctured, and humility is what comes of honesty: a realistic appraisal of who we really are. If we follow this with an honest desire to become who we can be, we are on our way to a life better than we ever imagined! Just how important is honesty? To us it is a vital matter in recovery and contented, useful living.

50.   PINK CLOUDS FULL OF LOVE AND HUGS
(Tongue in cheek)

Hi! My name is Muffin and I'm a grateful recovering alcoholic One Day at a Time by the Grace of God. What a miracle! I'm a walking miracle. Thank you, HP, for my miracle and allowing me to be part of others' miracles too. I've been a member of A.A. now for three months, and my heart is overflowing with gratitude for what all of you have given me each day, each meeting, each breath of freedom, and for all the friends and the friends I haven't met yet. I love A.A. and everyone in the Fellowship for all the caring and sharing. I especially like the hugs in A.A. which I learned to do in treatment.

Speaking of treatment, I'm still a little mad at Mother and Father, O.K., for sending me there. They really didn't send me there; they sort of tricked me. Oh! Maybe not quite tricked, but they didn't give me a chance to stop using by myself. If it wasn't for all those nice people in treatment, I probably would have left there.

I was introduced to those awesome 12 Steps in treatment, and I took the first five. Step 3 is my favorite. It was easy to "turn it over" to my HP.

At my meeting tonight I get my 3-month pin

and I asked Jeff to give it to me. He's sort of my sponsor; he sure knows a lot about the Program even if he's only been in 9 months. I'm sure glad I got rid of my other sponsor. You wouldn't believe the things she wanted me to do. I can't see any reason why she was so strict and bossy. Jeff is so much better and I think I have a crush on him. Wouldn't it be great if we started to see each other and go to meetings together all the time? Well, I got my hair and nails done and a new outfit for the meeting tonight.

I've got to go now, O.K., and read my sixty meditation books. I don't see why meditation is so hard to do with the help of my books, they're so full of LOVE. And I'd like to leave you with my favorite quote about hugs. Maybe I'll read it tonight at the meeting. Maybe we can sing the Serenity Prayers, too. Thanks for letting me share.

"Hugs are not only nice; they're needed. Hugs can relieve pain and depression, make the healthy healthier, the happy happier and the most secure among us even more so. Hugging feels good, overcomes fear, eases tension, provides stretching exercise if you're short and stooping exercise if you're tall. Hugging does not upset the environment, saves heat and requires no special equipment. It makes happy days happier and impossible days possible."

51.   OUR PAST
(4th and 5th Steps)

When we arrived in the Fellowship, we had a "past life" that we would just as soon forget. Some of us would wish all of it away; others just carefully selected events. And we were full of regrets; sometimes it seemed that the longer we were in the Program, the more regrets we had! We really wanted to run from the pain, humiliation, anger, fear, loneliness and feelings of inadequacy in our past. "Facing squarely up to it" was the *last* thing we wanted to do. The Fourth Step says, "Made a searching and fearless moral inventory of ourselves" (not others). And on top of that the Fifth Step says, "Admitted to God, to ourselves and to another human being the exact nature of *our* wrongs"! What painful suggestions! Why not just jump off a bridge and get it over with?

Relax, there is hope and promise for our future, if we are careful about our past. Those who've been here awhile tell us that we are only as Sick as Our Secrets. And that if we are thorough and omit nothing in these two Steps, we will be able to walk down the street with our heads held high living happy, useful lives. And there are some promises in the Big Book: *"We will not regret the past nor wish to shut the door on it. No matter how far down the scale we have gone, we will see how our experience can benefit others."*

Can you imagine? How could all of that mess in our past actually benefit others? If you've been around awhile and work with others, you already know the wonderful feeling associated with helping someone by sharing your own past. Sometimes sharing our past eases pain, defuses explosive situations or has a soothing effect on others. If you haven't been able to look at the past yet, "Keep coming back!" You are in for a miracle: a life with a brighter future, not a sordid past!

52.   GETTING OUT OF MYSELF
(Self-pity)

The Fifth Promise tells me "that feeling of uselessness and self-pity will disappear." I believe the Promises come as a direct result of ACTION, and the Fifth Promise materialized through my involvement in service work.

I have a disease of self-obsession, selfishness and self-centeredness. I became so wrapped up in how I felt, how I looked and how I was doing that I never had time for you. It never dawned on me that you had troubles, that you had feelings, that you needed me. Even in recovery it is easy for me to slide into a state where I am the sole center of the universe.

Thank heaven for sponsors! I was steered toward service work from the start: setting up before and cleaning up after meetings. I could not understand how doing "silly" things like that was going to make me feel better. My problems needed "deeper" treatment. It didn't dawn on me until some time later that my sponsor, in her wisdom, knew that when I was involved in the makings of a meeting, I didn't have time to think about myself. Through this interaction, I became aware of others in this universe besides me.

It is impossible to reach out to another person and also feel useless. It is impossible to try to help another person and feel sorry for yourself at the same time. When I am reaching out, I don't have time to worry about myself. And when I am alone again, I usually can't remember what I was torn up about, or it just doesn't seem that bad any more.

So the next time you feel mired in self-pity, ask yourself: "When was the last time I showed up at a meeting a half-hour early? When did I chair last? Clean up? Have I volunteered recently? When did I last take a newcomer to a meeting?"

53.   "IN A RELATIONSHIP"
(Sign of insecurity?)

During the past few years, I have heard much reference to a phenomenon commonly known as "being in a relationship." I have even been asked, on occasion, if I am "in a relationship." I have never known quite how to answer as I have never been quite sure what is meant by the phrase. Today, I decided to take a look in the dictionary and see if I could find any answers there.

Here are the observations I made after my trip through the *American Heritage Dictionary of the English Language*:

By definition a relationship only exists by reason of blood or marriage. Therefore, what are commonly referred to in our culture as "relationships" are not relationships at all. At best they are love affairs, though one must often use great imagination to find any evidence of love; and therefore they would probably most often fall into the category of a short or long form of sexual liaison.

It seems obvious that it requires two people in order to have a "relationship." However, I have heard individuals describing themselves as being "in a relationship" even though the other party denies its existence. As I see it, one person alone can make an emotional commitment to another; but there is no "relationship" without reciprocal commitments on the parts of two people.

I am inclined to think the phrase "in a relationship" was coined and is used by some of us who are so insecure within ourselves that we need to feel we are "in a relationship" when, indeed, we are not, or at least, we are afraid we are not.

I found it interesting that all definitions with reference to relationships are stated in the present tense, i.e., there is no connotation of them "going anywhere." It makes me wonder where the belief that relationships must go in some direction originated.

According to my understanding of the term, all relationships between people (other than those based on connection by blood or marriage), exist only as long as both parties are active participants by mutual agreement.

There is but one relationship always available to me, and that is with God because He has told me that I have to seek Him and He will be there, that He will never leave me nor forsake me. Human relationships based on real love can be patterned after this example of long-lasting commitment that God in His love has shown us. As each of us grows spiritually, the likelihood of our being able to receive and to give this type of loving commitment grows accordingly. As this happens, we simultaneously lose the need to know whether or not we are "in a relationship."

54.   JUST GO TO HIM

I hadn't been on my knees for long. A few minutes of a few twenty-four hours in a row. A few requests, a few pleas, a few sobs and lots of demands. I remember the early prayers. I couldn't think straight.

I didn't know what I was supposed to be asking for. I wasn't thinking that God loved me and that's why I was told to go to Him. I was thinking about me saving my own self. I was uncomfortable, no, I was freaked out about what God was going to do to me if I didn't shape up. I went to Him out of guilt, out of fear. I questioned my motives, my sincerity, my reasons for prayer. Did I really mean it? Did it really count? Was it good enough to warrant total and complete redemption? You know what I found out? He just wanted me to go to Him; just wanted me to do it. The rest? Well, He pretty much takes care of that.

55.   A FULL AND THANKFUL HEART

One exercise that I practice is to try for a full inventory of my blessings and then for a right acceptance of the many gifts that are mine, both temporal and spiritual. Here I try to achieve a state of joyful gratitude. When such a brand of gratitude is repeatedly affirmed and pondered, it can finally displace the natural tendency to congratulate myself on whatever progress I may have been enabled to make in some areas of living.

I try hard to hold fast to the truth that a full and thankful heart cannot entertain great conceits. When brimming with gratitude, one's heartbeat must surely result in outgoing love, the finest emotion that we can ever know.

56. HEARING A FIFTH STEP

I regret that within our literature there are no clear-cut directions for hearing someone else's Fifth Step. I heard my first Fifth before I did my own, and I got some valuable suggestions from my sponsor, such as: Pray, asking God how you can be helpful.

Review the first Three Steps and do the Third Step prayer together if they wish. Don't take on their stuff; let it go right on by. Share your own experiences and defects, if that is helpful. Listen for the "exact nature" of the wrongs, the fear, selfishness, dishonesty, etc., which is underneath the specific details, and write those down for the person to review at Steps 6 and 7. This writing also gives my head something to do, so I stay centered on the business at hand. Write down the people they may owe amends to if they want to destroy their Fourth Step. (I burned my first Fourth and felt set free by that symbolic act. I kept my second attempt and share it with people when that's helpful; lets them know they're not dealing with the Blessed Virgin!) If you hear minimizing, rationalizing or sliding over something, bring them back to look at what's being avoided.

Don't reveal anything shared during a Fifth Step. It is a vital confidence not to be broken. I have been privileged to hear many Fifth Steps.

I always learn something about me, and I

always feel closer to the person who's willing to share honestly. The two men whose Fifth Steps I have heard have taught me that men and women are not different in this disease: different words, same music, and the same fear, selfishness, and dishonesty. I basically hear Fifth Steps the way that mine was heard. It worked real well for me, and as we say, "If it ain't broke, don't fix it."

57.   PRESCRIPTION FOR SERENITY

No one ever gets out of this world alive. Resolve therefore to maintain a sense of values.

Take care of yourself. Good health is everyone's major source of wealth. Without it, serenity is harder to attain.

Resolve to be cheerful and helpful. People will repay in kind more often than not.

Avoid zealots. They are generally humorless.

Resolve to listen more and talk less. Rarely does anyone learn anything while talking.

Be wary of giving advice. The wise don't need it, and fools won't heed it.

Resolve to be tender with the young, compassionate with the aged, sympathetic with the striving, and tolerant of the weak and the wrong. Sometime in life you will have been all of these.

Do not equate money with success. The

world abounds with big money-makers who are miserable failures as human beings. What counts most about success is how a person achieves it.

Acknowledge lust when you feel it, but don't confuse it with love.

Don't take yourself too seriously. Humanity's saving grace is its sense of humor.

Set goals for yourself. Work hard to achieve them, but don't feel guilty if you don't. The hard work was your reward, not the achievement.

Learn to understand the Serenity Prayer: God grant me the serenity to accept the things I cannot change, the courage to change the things I can, and the wisdom to know the difference.

58.   STAYING BUSY
(God's will for me)

I was very active socially when I was using. By that, I mean I spent a lot of time in the various nightspots around town, enough to become known as a member of the regular crowd. I was always getting in the car with my girlfriend on any given night (it didn't matter if it was a work night), going to some bar or some party or SOMEWHERE, looking for action, looking for men, looking for excitement, always feeling restless, irritable and discontent. Whether I was happy or unhappy, I was always looking for something "more."

And it never seemed like enough. Maybe at first, for a couple of days or weeks, but eventually it got old or boring, and I felt terribly disillusioned. So I'd go on vainly looking for something "more."

I've found it very difficult at times to break out of this pattern of thinking in recovery. Turning my will and life over the care of God day by day is not always easy, and I still have a deep fear that God will not give me the things I think I need to be happy. I feel this fear and distrust particularly when I am going through spells of loneliness, depression, or self-pity.

I don't have a miracle answer or a wonderful sounding philosophy that will help me. But I have learned these things since coming to the Program: On my own I am nothing. I need God; I need willingness and action on my part by working the Steps; and I need hope that my fear will be removed. God's will not mine.

I know God has kept me abstinent for a while now and worked a lot of cleansing and healing in me. I've seen God do the same for so many people. I know the answer lies with Him and the Fellowship. I know that when I've gotten off my can and helped others through 12th Step work, I'M OKAY. I know that going to meetings regularly and sharing my real feelings makes me feel OKAY. I know that when I work the Steps I feel OKAY. I know that if I keep on praying and surrendering these old ideas I will continue to be OKAY.

And then maybe I'll suddenly realize that God has done for me what I could not do for myself, and thank Him.

59.   ON THE PITY POT

Am I on the pity pot? I hope not. I am in my fifth year, and I find recovery becoming more and more difficult. I have been without booze for a while; and I gave up cigarettes, a major feat! Now I have had to humble myself and go into another program to lose forty pounds.

My dysfunctional family was so angry and hostile toward me that I had to divorce them from my life. I am making major changes in relationships to take care of myself, and I find this difficult. I have always prided myself on getting along with everyone. And now, I am being forced to confront people, something that I hate to do. I never could express my anger; and now in order to survive in this world, I have to express my anger.

Beneath my anger is fear, and underneath my fear lies my insecurity. God, how can I admit this and make myself vulnerable?

"They" say that God gives us no more than we can bear. I feel that my Higher Power is pushing me too hard, but who am I to buck my Higher Power who knows me best of all! He is trying to show me some humility and courage so that I will change to be of some value to Him. After all, I now have a purpose in life one day at a time; and with His help and yours, I will humbly accept life's challenges as my chance to grow and to be more fruitful in our Fellowship and "out there"!

60.   UNMANAGEABLE
(Step 1)

For me the "unmanageable" part of the First Step is unquestionably true because things were in a constant state of disarray while I was using. The only thing that seemed manageable was the time I needed to indulge my habit; and I don't think I ever had trouble finding a spare hour or two, or three, or four, or ... to meet my objective.

After I admitted, through the help of my Higher Power, that I was powerless, I thought that everything would fall into place "nice, nice" and that now I would be able to enjoy living the second half of the First Step. Surely I'd be able to start managing my time now! I reasoned that with all the extra time on my hands I'd be able to do some of the things that I had put off for so long. Boy, I thought, *now* I can begin to start managing things! But, lo and behold, I found that I was mistaken because all of a sudden I had too many obligations and too many jobs to do, partially to right the wrongs I had done during my addiction and, yes, partially because, in spite of myself, my life was beginning to change -- for the better, I might add.

My house is still a mess sometimes. I'm still very impetuous. I still have trouble meeting deadlines. I still, on many occasions, allow *my* will to be my guiding force. I sometimes feel that "the hurrieder I go, the behinder I get." But, in spite of all the above, I do have a way to *handle* it now. The Program has given me the way to "cope."

61.   WORTH THE EFFORT
(Step 4)

I have some notions on the Fourth Step that I've gotten from doing meetings and a workshop on it, helping people through it, and studying it as a process. Since I want to share some of these ideas with you, and am not in on the workshop next month, I'm using this opportunity to do so.

Yes, I really mean "benevolent." At first, we all tend to see The Big Fourth as a scary, unforgiving, and unfinishable task. As we put it to good use, though, we find that the Fourth Step is a beneficial tool for recovery and serenity that we can use all our lives. Just as a written Fourth Step tells us enough about ourselves to get on with the whole Program, continuing the Fourth (few of us just do one) and living by it, as the

Twelfth urges us to do for all the Steps, helps us know and love ourselves enough to be truly useful, and therefore happy.

I think the Fourth Step scares us so much because what we fear most are our own darker instincts, urges, and fears, which many of us think of as "ourselves." Our desires and feelings are certainly part of us, but they don't control us, contrary to what many of us assumed (I sure did). We don't have to (and can't to stay sober) continue the ineffective over-reactions that let our instincts "dominate us" (quotes from here on are from the *12&12*) and that make up our "defects of character." The Fourth Step helps us change these patterns and let our true selves come out and "meet conditions, whatever they (are)."

I have yet to hear of anyone being harmed by doing or attempting any Fourth Step work. We even benefit from foggy attempts while in treatment. Since we're at the "beginning of a lifetime practice," we can start with "those flaws which are . . . troublesome and obvious" (do you have those, too?). Looking at resentments and our part of our relationships with people (as the Big Book suggests) makes sense, too, as it will uncover more of our problem areas and harm done. However we start, Fourth Steps always seem to work if we're honest and persistent.

It also pays to use all the help you can get. In careful doses, check in with people who really know you -- your sponsor, home group, friends and family. The ideas you need are in the many good recovery books. Fourth Step meetings and workshops did and do help me a lot, but remember to keep it simple and not get overloaded with ideas and recommendations (even these!).

I'm going to leave room for other good news. I hope this helps someone besides me get friendlier with the Fourth Step and with themselves! It may hurt a bit, but our real selves are worth the effort and worth knowing!

62.   THE BRIDGE TO CHANGE
(Humility)

I have learned from experience that staying abstinent and attending meetings through painful times is a guarantee of personality change. We no longer have to escape our pain through using. The Program has given us a precious tool which, used regularly, will transform pain into growth. Armed with humility, we who once dreaded change as much as death can learn to face real life with a new courage and hope.

During my using days, I lived in a fantasy world of my own creation. I attempted to control not only effort but outcomes of situations. I tried to keep myself calm with chemicals and food, with no recognition for the ups and downs of daily living. I was seeking an unreal world of complete security, romance and approval; and the more I tried to control (demand) these things, the more chaos I created. It becomes clear to us in getting sober that we have to change. I like what Bill Wilson has to say about these rude awakenings in this passage:

"As we grow spiritually, we find that our old attitudes toward our instinctual drives need to undergo drastic revisions. Our demands for emotional security and wealth, for personal prestige and power all have to be tempered and redirected. We learn that the full satisfaction of these demands cannot be the sole end and aim of our lives. We cannot place the cart before the horse, or we shall be pulled backward into disillusionment. But when we are willing to place spiritual growth first -- then and only then do we have a real chance to grow in healthy awareness and mature love." (Twelve & Twelve, p. 114)

Humility seems to be the basic ingredient for transforming pain into growth. In Step Seven of the Twelve & Twelve, humility is defined as the *"perspective to see that character-building and spiritual values have to come first, and that material satisfactions are not the purpose of living."* We learn that an honest desire to seek and do God's will is necessary for humility.

"What an order, I can't go through with it!" used to be my initial reaction to growing through the Steps. I could accept solutions intellectually, but when it came to practical application, I had trouble. I know today that I don't have to do it perfectly; it takes time to get better. I know that I don't have to do it alone; that I have a wealth of wisdom and support in this Fellowship at my disposal, and that gives me a lot of hope for changes, growth, and new frontiers.

63. A NEW BEGINNING
(Change)

The month of January is always a time of reflection for me. I dwell upon what I can see as change in myself and upon the shortcomings I still hold onto. I offer a passage from the story "Doctor, Alcoholic, Addict" which appears in the Big Book on pages 439-452.

"The people of A.A. had something that looked much better than what I had, but I was afraid to let go of what I had in order to try something new; there was a certain sense of security in the familiar.

"Now, what am I going to do about it? When I stopped living in the problem and began living in the answer, the problem went away. Acceptance is the answer to all my problems today. When I am disturbed, it is because I find some person, place, thing, or situation -- some fact of my life -- unacceptable to me, and I can find no serenity until I accept that person, place, thing, or situation as being exactly the way it is supposed to be at

this moment. Nothing, absolutely nothing happens in God's world by mistake. I need to concentrate not so much on what needs to be changed in the world as on what needs to be changed in me and in my attitudes."

Change began for me when I admitted and accepted the First Step: I am powerless over alcohol and my life is unmanageable. The power to accomplish this change comes from the first word of the First Step: WE, a word that freed me from the isolated loneliness of addiction. Because the Fellowship of AA existed I am able to enjoy the benefits of a sober lifestyle. To recover implies a process of change, sometimes intentional and sometimes not intentional. If you attend meetings, meetings, meetings, the AA Program will work its magic upon you by exposure. AA is the key which released me from a hell of misery and pain. This past Thanksgiving I attended the Inspiration Group at St. Barnabas Church and heard Glenn S. say, "Alcohol wasn't my problem. Alcohol was my solution. My problem was me." It certainly was my solution. My problem is most definitely me. Alcohol and drugs allowed me to escape. It colored my world with illusions and delusions of my own making. Reality, or what I thought was reality, was a fantasy. Reality, for me now, means making sobriety priority #1, while learning to live one day at a time with the me that is. Recovery and change are made so much easier by having a spiritual basis for life. As it states in the Big

Book: *"If a mere code of morals or a better philosophy
of life were sufficient to overcome alcoholism, many of
us would have recovered long ago. Lack of power, that
was our dilemma. We had to find a power by which we
could live, and it had to be a power greater than ourselves."* I would like to close with two more passages
taken from the Big Book on pages 103 and 164.

> *"After all, our problems were of our own making.
Bottles were only a symbol. Besides, we have stopped
fighting anybody or anything. We have to.*

> *"Abandon yourself to God as you understand
God. Admit your faults to Him and to your fellows.
Clear away the wreckage of your past. Give freely of what
you find and join us. We shall be with you in the
Fellowship of the Spirit, and you will surely meet some
of us as you trudge the Road of Happy Destiny.*

> *May God bless you and keep you -- until then."*

64.   COUNTING OUR BLESSINGS

Count your garden by the flowers,
Never by the leaves that fall.
Count your days by golden hours,
Don't remember clouds at all.
Count your nights by stars, not shadows,
Count your life by smiles, not tears.
And with joy on every birthday,
Count your age by friends, not years.

65. SLOGANS

1. Easy Does It
2. First Things First
3. Live and Let Live
4. But for the Grace of God
5. Think ... Think ... Think
6. One Day at a Time
7. Let Go and Let God
8. K.I.S.S. - Keep It Simple Stupid
9. Act As If ...
10. This Too Shall Pass
11. Expect A Miracle
12. I Can't ... God Can ... I Think I'll Let Him
13. If It Works ... Don't Fix It
14. Keep Coming Back ... It Works If You Work It
15. Stick With the Winners
16. Identify Don't Compare
17. Recovery Is A Journey, Not A Destination
18. Faith Without Works Is Dead
19. Poor Me ... Poor Me ... Pour Me Another Drink
20. To Thine Own Self Be True
21. I Came; I Came To; I Came To Believe
22. Live In The NOW

23. If God Seems Far Away, Who Moved?
24. Turn It Over
25. Utilize, Don't Analyze
26. Nothing Is So Bad, A Drink Won't Make It Worse
27. We Are Only As Sick As Our Secrets
28. There Are No Coincidences In The Program
29. Be Part Of The Solution, Not The Problem
30. Sponsors: Have One - Use One - Be One
31. I Can't Handle It God; You Take Over
32. Keep An Open Mind
33. It Works--It Really Does!
34. Willingness Is The Key
35. More Will Be Revealed
36. You Will Intuitively Know
37. You Will Be Amazed
38. No Pain . . . No Gain
39. Go For It
40. Principles Before Personalities
41. Do It Sober
42. Let It Begin With Me
43. Just For Today
44. Sober 'n Crazy
45. Pass It On
46. It's In The Book
47. You Either Is--Or You Ain't

48.   Before You Say: I Can't . . . Say: I'll Try
49.   Don't Quit 5 Minutes Before The Miracle
        Happens
50.   Some Of Us Are Sicker Than Others
51.   We're All Here Because We're Not All There
52.   Addiction Is An Equal Opportunity Destroyer
53.   Practice An Attitude Of Gratitude
54.   The Road To Recovery Is A Simple Journey
        For Confused People With A Complicated
        Disease
55.   Another Friend Of Bill W's
56.   God Is Never Late
57.   Have A Good Day Unless You've Made Other
        Plans
58.   Shit Happens
59.   It Takes Time
60.   90 Meetings 90 Days
61.   You Are Not Alone
62.   Wherever You Go, There You Are
63.   Don't Drink, Read The Big Book, And Go To
        Meetings
64.   Use The 24-Hour Plan
65.   Make Use Of Telephone Therapy
66.   Stay Sober For Yourself
67.   Look For Similarities Rather Than
        Differences

68.   Remember Your Last Drunk
69.   Remember That Alcoholism Is Incurable,
       Progressive, and Fatal
70.   Try Not To Place Conditions On Your
       Recovery
71.   When All Else Fails Follow Directions
72.   Count Your Blessings
73.   Share Your Happiness
74.   Respect The Anonymity of Others
75.   Share Your Pain
76.   Let Go Of Old Ideas
77.   Try To Replace Guilt With Gratitude
78.   What Goes Around, Comes Around
79.   Change Is A Process, Not An Event
80.   Take The Cotton Out Of Your Ears And Put
       It In Your Mouth
81.   Call Your Sponsor Before, Not After, You
       Take The First Drink
82.   Sick And Tired Of Being Sick And Tired
83.   It's The First Drink That Gets You Drunk
84.   To Keep It, You Have To Give It Away
85.   Man's Extremity Is God's Opportunity
86.   The Price For Serenity And Sanity Is
       Self-sacrifice
87.   One Alcoholic Talking To Another

66.   CO-DEPENDENCY: AN INTIMACY DILEMMA
(By Sondra Smalley, CCDP, Licensed Psychologist)

> *"It don't matter to me,*
> *if you take up with someone*
> *who's better than me,*
> *'cuz your happiness is all I want*
> *for you to find . . ."*
>   David Gates
>   "It Don't Matter to Me"

We all want to belong in this world. We want to belong and feel useful in the world of work, in social situations and in close relationships. Alfred Adler, a psychiatrist who did extensive studies of people's relationships, thought that many of us become discouraged because we don't feel that we belong, even as young children. It has been suggested that from this pursuit of belonging, co-dependent patterns emerge.

Co-dependency is a term used to describe an exaggerated dependent pattern of learned behaviors, beliefs and feelings that make life painful. It is a dependence on people and things outside the self along with neglect of the self to the point of having little self-identity.

It is not particular to a specific age group, type of relationship, or gender.

The following questions and answers are reprinted from a taped interview with Sondra Smalley about the scope and nature of the intimacy dilemma.

Sondra Smalley has been doing extensive work in the area of relational concerns. Smalley has her master's degree in counseling and psychological services, is a private counselor, and has over 20 years' experience in the helping professions.

Question: Is there something wrong with dependency?

Answer: No, all relationships have inter-dependencies. We are talking about extreme or exaggerated dependencies.

Question: What are some signs or symptoms that people could look for in themselves to help determine if they might have co-dependent tendencies?

Answer: People could ask themselves a number of questions. First, is my life in balance physically, mentally, emotionally, and spiritually; or am I neglecting myself and concentrating on other people, other things, others' problems?

Do I know who I am? Do I have a clear identity? Do I know who I am apart from the roles I play?

Am I satisfied with my friendships? Do I have

as many friends as I want and what is the quality of those relationships?

Am I satisfied with my work? Does it meet my need for being productive?

Am I satisfied with my intimate relationships? Do I know how to be intimate without fusion or isolation?

Ask yourself if you are generally satisfied with your life. If not, look for threads of connection throughout your relationship history. There would be cause for concern if there is a history of unsatisfying relationships without an understanding of the causes of the dissatisfaction.

A key is: are you good to yourself? Are you gentle with yourself, or do you tend to neglect yourself? The reasons are not important. Often, co-dependent people will rationalize neglecting themselves because they are too busy taking care of or worrying about others. Behind this is the belief that love is defined by being responsible FOR others.

Question: What is the significance of that?

Answer: Without realizing it, these people are choosing to be externally controlled. They are other-directed and find it hard to be their own person. They often think or feel or say, "I don't care," "it doesn't matter to me" or "I'm happy if they are." They try to be loving and caring by being responsible FOR others. This caretaking role is usually very frustrating.

A more comfortable way to be is responsible TO one's self and TO others.

Question: What are the differences between being responsible FOR others and being responsible TO others?

Answer: People who are responsible FOR others tend to be concerned with answers, solutions, being right, details, performance and mistakes.

People who are responsible to themselves and to others tend to be concerned with relating to others, caring, being compassionate, being "okay" to themselves and to others.

Co-dependents often feel anxious, discouraged, fearful, used, put upon, depressed, self-neglectful and tense instead of feeling comfortable, calm and peaceful.

Question: How easy is it to recognize?

Answer: That really is hard to say. Co-dependents tend to carry or store their feelings. They do things like manipulate, project blame, intellectualize, minimize, protect, fix, control, deny feelings and rescue. Characteristics of people who act responsible to themselves and to others do things like empathize, confront, level, share feelings and assert.

When co-dependents take responsibility for others, they are cancelling them out and taking from them opportunities to take care of themselves. This makes everyone anxious and preoccupied about the outcome. It takes a lot of time and energy to be responsible for others. It requires one to spend less time taking care of the self. Being responsible to yourself and to others allows both people to live their own lives, respecting each other, caring about what is happening and being supportive.

Question: Does being responsible FOR others play a major role in co-dependent behavior?

Answer: Definitely. Co-dependents think, "if I love somebody, I must be concerned with finding solutions for his/her life."

This brings up another question you can ask yourself when you're in a relationship. "Am I concerned with the other person doing the right thing rather than a general concern for that person's 'okayness'?"

Question: Could you give an example?

Answer: Hypothetically, a co-dependent person is what I call the "supermom." She has a career and a family. She comes home from work, walks in the door and says, "Whose car is in the driveway? Why aren't the dishes done? Did you go to the dentist today? Were you on time for school? Get your feet off the coffee table." Her sense of responsibility is overwhelming. There is such preoccupation and concentration of being the caretaker that there is no mutual respect in the relationship.

Question: What happens to the supermom

when the last child grows up and leaves home?

Answer: Often there are love shifts, where the people being taken care of are changed. There may be depression, or possibly her days or evenings will be filled with outside activities such as dancing, softball, bowling, etc. The problem is that there are no self-rewards in these activities. They are merely ways of keeping busy. There may also be total self-neglect.

Question: Self-neglect in what way?

Answer: Things such as not going to the doctor. Not going to the dentist. Not spending money on herself. Giving up close friends, hobbies or passing up opportunities that would make her happy.

Question: Is there a rationalization for not doing things that are self-rewarding?

Answer: Yes, and this involves most co-dependents, not just the supermoms. Co-dependents are often no longer able to know what satisfies them. They completely lose touch and are not clear about what makes them happy. They often are not even sure of who they are. They tend to see themselves only in the role of mother, child, spouse, friend, salesperson, etc., and cannot answer the question, "Who am I?"

They also tend to wonder about things such as, "Who should I be like so that people will like me?" They are not comfortable or are not able to just present themselves to others.

Question: What are the consequences of co-dependency?

Answer: Depression, physical symptoms, stress-related illnesses which come from always living a very tense life, always trying to be externally directed. Practicing impression management, which is a term used to describe adjusting your behavior in order to control what other people think of you. This would include watching everything that you do, say, what you wear, a complete monitoring of the self so that there is absolute control over how you are perceived

Co-dependents are often spectators in life. There is usually no true intimacy in their relationships. They may believe that they have a lot of friends, but people rarely get to know them. They do, however, get to know others rather well because of their tendency toward being very observant people.

Question: What distinguishes the co-dependent person from a person who may just have some symptoms of co-dependency?

Answer: One major symptom is self-neglect. Co-dependents do not take good care of themselves. Are the activities they are involved in rewarding or just plain physically and emotionally exhausting? Is there an overall feeling of satisfaction or a feeling of always being on edge?

Question: So, in addition to the self-neglect, the co-dependent keeps busy for the purpose of not thinking?

Answer: Yes. In a lot of cases, the co-dependent is in a "zombie" state. They report not feeling much of anything. They are not usually very concerned with this lack of feeling, but view it as a curiosity. They just do not feel different over time as opposed to the hundreds of ways that people can feel.

Question: Is it a feeling of "everything's fine"?

Answer: Yes, but this usually happens along with the feeling of responsibility.

Question: What's a typical pattern for co-dependents when going into a new relationship?

Answer: They tend to be highly tolerant, to hide what they truly want to do, or what one wants or needs from a relationship, a real high involvement in impression management, as well as a tendency to be concerned with the person's demeanor and behavior being proper.

Question: Will that other person detect something?

Answer: Yes, usually the other person will just go away. They may not want to be taken care of, or have the co-dependent person assume responsibility for him/her.

Question: Then it is an extreme; the co-dependent person will start out acting either aloof and controlled or totally smothering?

Answer: Right. Usually one extreme or the

other, but often aloof at first and then when those walls come tumbling down, there's fusion. Here again, there are things people can ask themselves. "Do I try to be more mature, more together than I really feel? Do I smile when I am angry or sad, or just have a general tendency for what I feel on the inside to not match what I show on the outside?"

There is also a very high tolerance for inappropriate behavior. Co-dependent people are very, very tolerant of behavior that other people would often ask, "How can you put up with that?"

Question: Is this an outer tolerance rather than a felt inner tolerance?

Answer: Yes, it is usually tolerance directed by impression management. Usually people's self-images are all tied up with being all-caring, all-giving, almost a perfectionist image of the self with ideals so extreme that they can't possibly be that way. Along with this are denial and excuses: denial of reality and excuses for inappropriate behavior. Also, there is a tendency to hold onto excuses for why life isn't perfect.

Question: Are there stages of co-dependency?

Answer: Oh definitely. In fact, the symptoms, for the most part, that I have been talking about are in the Phase I stage. I divide co-dependency into two stages, Phases I and II.

Question: What happens in Phase II?

Answer: The most serious sign I look for is a tremendous focus on outside activities in concurrence with extreme under-responsibility for the self. These people keep busy until they drop, from PTA to golf to church to softball--whatever.

Question: And these activities contain no self-pleasure?

Answer: Right. These activities are used to alleviate the person of thinking or concentrating on the self. If they are busy until they fall exhausted into bed at night, there isn't much time for introspection. People also start having tolerance breaks in this stage and go into rages. They're very over-reactive and deal with almost any unpleasant situation by raging.

The tendency to cope is pretty much gone by now. These people have also adopted some very rigid attitudes. They may have even started reading books trying to figure out for themselves what the problem is. They're smart people, and they have all the answers; they just don't know what the questions are. They also tend to do a lot of comparison of themselves with others; they observe what others do right and copy them.

At this stage, co-dependents often become so discouraged in trying to relate that they simply give up.

Question: Do many people get this far?

Answer: It's hard to say for sure, but I would guess that one fourth of the people may, at least in people 50 years and under.

Question: What does the recovery process involve?

Answer: The first step involves getting people to look at themselves and see what is on the inside. I suggest people begin to view change as a learning process, not a test.

Question: Such as . . . ?

Answer: First, know thyself. Learn how to trust the center within you. The second step involves the belief that change is possible. Then, having the courage of hope, people begin to engage in small changes of behavior. The key words here are small changes, and also accepting failures as part of the process. The main goal is to have introspection focusing on the self without guilt. I have specific ideas that I give to people to begin this process. Also included here is stopping observation of others and stopping the impression management. One method I use is having the people keep journals with very specific assignments given to help keep them self-focused.

The next step would be spontaneous introspection along with examination of who that person is in relationship to others. Looking at their history, have they always been victims in relationships?

Question: Why is it important for co-dependents to go back to looking at who they are in relationship to others?

Answer: Because if there is little self-identity, and one goes to bond with another person, there will likely be fusion. Without a defined "self-identity" and understanding of the self in terms of others, the self takes on a chameleon-like role who guesses what the other wants him/her to be. Co-dependent people tend to have a hard time saying, "I want." Most co-dependents feel that others can define who they are better than they can. They know the roles that they are; they just don't know *who* they are.

Question: What are your suggestions for people to begin the process of making small changes?

Answer: Finding others who care. Developing a network of friends who are also changing co-dependent patterns. This is important because they will understand and relate to the feelings, attitudes and behaviors being experienced.

Begin focusing on the present, observing what is going on now. The past is important only if it relates to the present, or as a means to detect a history of co-dependent patterns. These patterns of feelings, behaviors and beliefs can be unlearned and replaced.

Learn to judge decisions according to the value they have for you. This involves understanding that meaningfulness comes from forming and living up to one's personal standards.

Plan successes. Many co-dependents have very high unrealistic expectations for themselves. This tends to always result in failure. It is important to plan little successes that are specific and simple, but achievable.

Do not justify failures. Failures are failures. They're no big deal. Don't analyze them; don't spend lots of time figuring out why things didn't go as planned. It's important to learn not to focus on failures.

Lastly, decrease self-punishment. Everyone makes mistakes. No one deserves to be punished because something did not work out. Punishment in this form of worry, shame, or guilt is the result of believing that you must be punished. A concept I use is that "we are learning to be gentle but firm with ourselves."[1]

(Based on an interview with Sondra Smalley by Jill Willis.)

67.   LIFE IS FAIR
(Step 11)

Often I hear someone say, "I don't know a thing," or, "The longer I'm in recovery the less I know." As a newcomer I found this frightening, but the longer I am in recovery the more I disagree with these statements. One never learns less! The more I learn, the more I realize I know only a little.

I often hear that life is not "fair." I believe

that life is always fair. It's my perception of it that is not.

My body never lies to me. That innermost self always seems to know. If only I could convince my head to trust those feelings. My body always knows the truth.

This is the only moment in which I can live, right now; there is no other time. Through practicing the Eleventh Step, I am able to experience the love and peace of being with myself and allowing the God of my understanding to flow through every cell of my body. Through practicing being in this moment, I can experience life in the now. Through practicing being in the moment, I can enjoy the fullness of where I am, always; don't miss it.

Knowing how to climb up the stairs does not get me to the top. The action I take may get me to the top, but if I rush or jump over some of the steps, I may fall. I find that taking them one at a time, one right after another, I will get where I want to go.

68.   I DIDN'T KNOW I DIDN'T KNOW
(I'm the problem)

The longer I'm in recovery, the more I keep finding out that I don't know what I know.

When I first came to the Program, there were a lot of things I thought I knew. My delusions of life, and especially of self, had told me that I was almost an expert on just about any given subject. My expertise included education, employment situations, love, relationships, sex, marriage, children, religion, etc.

Ironically, these were the very things that I felt so sorry for myself about. I had had all these people, places, and things; but for some strange reason, certainly not me, I no longer had any of them. I believed that I was a victim of this cruel and unfair world.

Gradually, over my years in recovery, I have gotten a second chance to learn about reality and self. One by one, I have been given back all the people, places and things that I traded away for my addiction. It's strange that I didn't get any of them back until I was ready to admit that I knew absolutely nothing about dealing with them.

My tendency was still to run or blame, but thanks to this wonderful Program, I have learned that "I am the problem." I still have the same choices as before, but this time I am choosing to learn by asking for help and feeling the pain. Pain really is growth fertilizer for me.

I came to the Program for help with my addiction, but I have been given so much more. Today, I know that "I didn't know I didn't know," and now that I know I don't know, it's perfectly O.K.

69.   A MEMBER'S MEDITATION ON STEP NINE

Have you thanked someone today, your H.P., your family, your friends, your fellow members ?

I heard someone remark at a Step meeting recently (re: Step Nine) that making amends, to them, meant making changes. We may not be able to change the past, but the present is within our reach to let certain individuals know that we are sorry, but also grateful for their patience, their time, their understanding. I think that gratitude is a positive element in making amends.

In meditating upon Step Nine, I realize I want to say: "I am sorry, but I want to change; and I appreciate you for investing in me your time, your patience, your understanding, and for seeing in me someone worthwhile. I am sorry for the past, but I will try to change for the better and am grateful for the opportunity!"

70.   RESENTMENT/POISON

Resentment is a deadly poison that seems to plague us all at times, even after some time in recovery.

It is a problem that will no doubt plague us most of our lives. The Program does try to help us become aware of its dangers.

The Program has taught me that:

1. Resentment robs me of serenity.
2. Resentment makes happiness impossible.
3. Resentment uses up energy that could go to accomplishment.
4. Resentment can become an emotional habit, making us habitually feel that we are victims of injustice.
5. Resentment is an emotional re-hashing of some event or circumstance of the past. You can't win because you can't change the past.
6. Resentment is not caused by other persons, circumstances, or events, but by our own emotional responses.

One way to handle resentment is to decide how much resentment the person, circumstance, or event deserves (which is very little), or how much I want to suffer. With resentment, like anger, nobody suffers but me.

Then I have to say to myself, "Who needs it!" and call someone in the Program and go to a meeting.

71.   WORKING FOR THE GOOD THINGS

Would life be worth it if it were easy? I think not. Too many times we are given things we don't have to work for. When we were young, a lot of times all we had to do was just ask for a toy or a new dress and they were given to us. Usually what happened was the toy got broken out of disregard, and the dress got torn out of neglect. It really didn't matter, for we knew we could ask for another one.

I feel that when we work for things that are very dear and special to us, they seem to be just a little more special to us. If life were easy, wouldn't we miss out on a few things? For example, if all we had were good times, would we appreciate them as much as if we never had a bad time to judge it by? I think not. Would we ever know freedom from bondage if we never had self-pity? I think not. Would we ever know serenity if we never had a day of turmoil? I think not.

I feel that all good things must be worked and striven for. If not, they wouldn't really mean much to us. We have to let God do for us what we can't do for ourselves.

72. EGO -- GOOD VS. BAD

Ego isn't all bad. We sometimes get that impression in meetings. Ego can be a motivation to achieve, and if it is for the good of the Program as a whole, then how can it be considered a character defect?

In my case, it becomes a defect when I am right and the rest of you "out there" don't know what you are talking about. "No one understands me." That, I have come to realize, is my warning signal; my EGO has taken over. It is time for me to find a quiet place and do some soul-searching. And what I usually come up with is balance; or as the dictionary says, *"emotional equilibrium, a harmonious or satisfying arrangement."* My ego returns to normal, and you out there aren't nearly as goofy as I thought you were.

What I guess I am trying to say is: life will always be a struggle with our ego, but we can keep it manageable, if we ask ourselves the question, "Is it to make me look good, or will it benefit others more?"

73. WHERE AM I?

Where am I with you, God, right now? I think it's a good question to ask from time to time. I think prayer is fine, but I should stop and listen and not do all the talking. I also find that praying out loud helps. You already know what I need; I need to hear myself say it.

I am finding that the Serenity Prayer is meaning more to me now. In my natural state, I am a "head-banger" (my own, that is) against the psychological walls I make when things don't go my way. Even saying the word SERENITY gives me some. The Serenity Prayer reminds me that I am powerless over many things and that I should release these matters to my Higher Power. The problems I can do something about, maybe, I should discuss with my Higher Power and possibly my sponsor first and LISTEN. It's easy for my self-will to run riot, even in recovery.

God, you knew my stubbornness; and in the beginning I saw You only through other people, their kind words, hugs, acceptance and the changes in their lives. I looked at them in amazement. I could not deny what I was seeing. It's been a very gradual process; but sometimes when I stop to listen, I hear a voice coming from within, giving me the reassurance I need.

74. PUTTING THE PROGRAM TO DAILY USE
(Step 10)

Step 10: *Continued to take personal inventory and when we were wrong promptly admitted it.*

Today I am looking at the Steps as 12 Steps going up which I had to climb one at a time (no escalator) after fighting my addiction for so long.

For me, they consisted of something like this: Steps 1, 2 and 3--Give up. Stop fighting this battle and surrender. Become a winner. Steps 4, 5 and 6--Open up. Be willing to look at myself, and share with another person and God all the things I had been using alcohol to avoid. Be willing to give them up. Steps 7, 8 and 9-- Ask God to help me get rid of these defects and shortcomings. Make up. Make amends to people I had harmed.

The first nine Steps were preparing me for a new way of life.

Approaching Step 10, I began to put my new way of living into practical use day by day. By this time in my recovery and journey to a better way of life, my house is in order. All the trash in my life has been sacked and is gone to the dump. I am no longer having hangovers. Here comes the real test: emotional hang-overs. These come as a direct result of my excesses of negative emotions: fear, anger, jealousy, etc. When I don't feel good about myself, I first have to examine my behavior today.

Is my behavior harmful for someone, either directly or indirectly? Most likely it is. I sometimes speak or act too quickly and don't think these through. Until I can go to the person and admit I am wrong, I cannot find peace again. I am not always able to do this promptly because I still tend to avoid pain.

Once I have done this, I am free again to enjoy this new way of life.

What about "justifiable" anger? If someone hurts me, don't I have a right to be angry? My program tells me to turn this over to someone better qualified to handle it. If I try to do this by myself, I will set myself up to fall into an emotional booby-trap. All I need to do is be willing to forgive if the fault lies elsewhere. Each day I must continue to sack up the trash in my life and send it to the dumping place.

Nothing is going to happen today which God and the principles of this Program will not help me to resolve. I can go back anytime to the Step I need to apply for any situation.

75.   "I DIDN'T HAVE TIME"

I got up early one morning
And rushed right into the day;
I had so much to accomplish
That I didn't have time to pray.
Problems just tumbled about me
And heavier came each task;
"Why doesn't God help me," I wondered.
He answered, "You didn't ask."
I wanted to see joy and beauty

But the day toiled on, gray and bleak.
I wondered why God didn't show me.
He said, "But you didn't seek."
I tried to come into God's presence;
I used all my keys at the lock.
God gently and lovingly chided,
"My child, you didn't knock."
I woke up early this morning
And paused before entering the day.
I had so much to accomplish
That I had to take time to pray.

76. BLAME AS A BLOCK TO RECOVERY

As long as I blame others, circumstances, and past events for my present situation, I am not accepting my own responsibility; and therefore, no growth or change can occur.

Blame is the way we humans shrug off responsibility for things occurring in our lives. By continually blaming, I refuse to look at the contributions my behaviors make to the situation; and therefore, I do nothing to change. As I give reason after reason for things not going the way I like, I keep myself from looking inward and choosing what I can do to change whatever is making me unhappy. Even laying guilt trips on my parents, spouse, or children does nothing to really alter my unhappiness. I have adapted to living with someone who has consistently disappointed, humiliated, angered and disgusted me. I have blamed, cajoled, supported, and defended the chemically dependent. I have questioned my judgment in choosing to remain in contact with a person who is "weak" and simultaneously I have feared my own inadequacies. I have rationalized my relationship with that person just as she has rationalized using.

Blaming another keeps me a slave; I am helpless in another's hands as my feelings become the responsibility of someone else. I will never be in charge of my own person if I choose to turn that control (blame) over to another. Blaming closes me to feedback because I rationalize why I am "right" and the other is "wrong," and I choose not to listen to what I label as "wrong."

If another is blamed for, or accepts responsibility for, my failures, then that person must also be credited for my successes, and vice versa, and this reduces that individual to non-personhood.

The only way to get out of this trap is to stop blaming. I refuse to let myself complain, find fault, or accuse another for my frustrations, sadness, and lack of a satisfying lifestyle. This process will take effort and practice, for old habits are difficult to break; but once I recognize that blaming another keeps me from participating wholly in life, I will find that my family, friends, and others close to me will help restore me to sanity. (One suggestion for working on new behaviors is to announce that I wish to get rid of this shortcoming and that I want those around me to signal me when I fall in the trap again.)

I know that every new bit of growth takes effort and concentration until it becomes a part of my life. Relationships don't get better in and of themselves. It takes commitment and effort. Communications long couched in mutual blame-laying must be replaced with the ability to say how I feel and to accept responsibility for my feelings without laying the cause of them on another. By using "I" in stating my thoughts, sensory experience, feelings, intentions, and actions, instead of "You," "We," and "Us," I take responsibility for myself and allow others to take responsibility for themselves.

Before I can accept my powerlessness in dependency, as the dependent or co-dependent, I need to eliminate blame from my thoughts, attitude, and communications. Only then will I be able to be responsible in my relationships.

Responsibility, then, is the ability to fulfill my needs, and to do this in a way that does not deprive others of the ability to fulfill their needs.

77.   WHEN ALL ELSE FAILS, FOLLOW DIRECTIONS

Why is recovery so difficult for some and seemingly easy for others? Like a woman who uses a new recipe, and wonders why the dish wasn't as good as the woman's next door, she may find that the directions are simple, but she can foul it up easily if directions are not followed.

One of the directions in the Program is, "Don't get on the wagon, get on the Program." The Program directs you simply: first be honest with yourself, no more games, alibis, lies, or false promises! If you are honest with yourself, you can then turn your problems over to the Higher Power. This first direction is repeated over and over again, and yet many fail to follow the first direction.

The next direction is to lay out a program for addiction-free daily living. Next comes involving yourself in a Program seeking to help others seeking recovery. It is said that ours is a simple Program and the directions are easy to follow; but somehow too many try short-cuts, substitutions, and like the woman with the new recipe, discover they substituted some ingredient or left out an important step. So again remember KISS: "Keep it simple, stupid." And when all else fails, follow directions.

78.   TEN COMMANDMENTS OF HUMAN RELATIONS

1. **Speak to people**. There is nothing as nice as a big cheerful word of greeting.

2. **Smile at people**. It takes 72 muscles to frown and only 14 to smile.

3. **Call people by name**. The sweetest music to anyone's ear is the sound of their own name.

4. **Be friendly and helpful**. If you would have friends, be friendly.

5. **Be cordial**. Speak and act as if everything you do is a genuine pleasure.

6. **Be generous with praise and cautious with criticism.**

7. **Be thoughtful of the opinions of others**. There are three sides to a controversy: yours, the other person's and the right one.

8. **Be alert to give service**. What counts most in life is what we do for others.

9. **Be genuinely interested in people**. You can like almost everyone if you try.

10. **Be considerate of the feelings of others.**

79.   I DON'T GO TO MEETINGS ANYMORE

First off, I'm a female alcoholic, and I owe a year and a half of happy sobriety to the desperate telephone call made to the A.A. telephone number. I still think that A.A. is a wonderful organization, although I no longer attend meetings.

Making the decision to call for help was the first step up out of the suicidal slime, and if there had been no A.A. to call I might never have made it. I'd already tried psychiatry with no success. Tranquilizers didn't seem the answer. Trying to stop drinking, with all one's friends and relatives still imbibing freely, though not as persistently, seemed impossible. Apparently, however, A.A. succeeds through group therapy; unfortunately the same group that I am now going to criticize very cruelly.

Most of my criticism has no doubt been voiced countless times, and probably there is no real solution. The trouble is mainly the people belonging to local A.A. groups, and who can do anything about people? My only aim in writing is to convey the thought that many hopeful alcoholics may be discouraged and drop out of A.A., back into their private hells, when the first happy relief of not drinking passes and they take a cold sober look at their comrades. I was disillusioned and just stopped going to the meetings. I had received the message, however. Just the thought of that horrible other me kills any desire for drink. I pray God it will always be so.

The two charming ladies who called on me that portentous May afternoon (after I dialed the number I'd been debating for so long) were the best of friends, I supposed. This pretense was maintained for at least a week, when I found to my surprise that they hated each other's guts.

Then a concerted effort was made by one group to unseat one of my sponsors from her chairmanship. Failing this, the conspirators started a new meeting on the same night of the week, which caused considerable controversy in all other groups: "That's pretty good--people who haven't been dry six months starting new meetings." If I seemed confused by all this bickering within the supposed serenity, someone said, "You should have been here back in such-and-such a year--this is nothing."

Or someone would phone and say, "So-and-so says you're not going to enough meetings!" I have three preteen kids who need their new improved mother at home in the evening. "So-and-so said this and that, and I'm so mad I could go get drunk." Children breaking their toys? "Well, everyone got through the holidays okay except for you-know-who, but then she welcomes any excuse." Is each holiday a fresh emergency to check the casualties? Almost every meeting produced some idiotic debate such as "Is it permissible to drink sweet cider?" Once a bunch of drunks came to the door of a meeting creating a disturbance. Everyone laughed. True, probably you can't help them in that condition, but *laugh*? *Us*?

I met women who were neglecting their children by attending meetings nightly, in town, out of town, anniversary, Al-Anon, speaking engagements, etc. Isn't that a substitution for the liquor that separated them from their obligations before? Another thing: I attended A.A. get-togethers off and on for nearly a year and saw only one black person. Is there segregation in A.A., or don't black people have any drinking problems?

In another vein, why is there so little actual anonymity? Someone might get up to speak, giving only his first name, but everyone appeared to know not only his last name, but how many times he'd been married and how much he still owed on his car.

And how some of them love to get up and talk. Disappointed thespians all, and how tiresome it gets! And how hideous when it's you standing up there, trying to avoid dredging up the waste products of your past and wishing you'd stayed home. I liked the round-table discussions best where coffee was served as the talk went on, but I suppose they can't do that all the time.

I know I met some fine, sincere people in
A.A., some I would have liked to know better. Perhaps
I let the petty personalities blind me to the organization as a whole. I'd love to help someone else who
needs it as I did, but would hesitate to introduce the
quaking, fearful, but still hopeful creature to that
assembly that met almost directly over the beer joint,
whose lively jukebox was clearly audible through the
uninspiring speeches and the after-coffee-and-dough-
nut gossip. To quote my former pals, "It almost made
you want to get drunk."

This won't do any good, but it's something
I've wanted to say for a long time, and I feel better.[2]

80.   GRACE

I asked for the grace to give,
to share, to console another,
to dress a hurting wound,
to lift a fallen spirit,
to mend a quarrel,
to dismiss a suspicion and replace it with trust,
to encourage someone who has lost faith,
to search out a forgotten friend,
to let someone feeling helpless do a favor for me,
to keep a promise,
to reduce my demands on others,

to fight for a principle,
to express gratitude,
to appreciate the beauty of nature,
to overcome a fear,
to forgive a hurt,
to tell someone I love them,
and then tell them again.

81.   YOU'RE THE MOST IMPORTANT PERSON HERE TONIGHT

When I attended my first meeting, a grandfatherly man acting as chairperson looked at me and said, "You're the most important person here tonight."

Well, that statement was just what I liked to hear, because I throve on attention. I went home from the meeting that night and thought long and hard. Two nights later, at the next meeting, I went in feeling very sure that I was still the most important person there. As a matter of fact, for the first thirty days or so, I felt I was doing the rest of the group a favor just by coming to their meetings!

We have a fairly small group and don't see many newcomers daily. But eventually, when another newcomer did make their way through the doors and

the chairperson called them the most important person in attendance that night, I was confused and hurt.

Today, I understand what that expression
means: without new people, we'd have no members at
all. Everyone has to come for the first time! I'd had
another wrong notion: once the "youngest" (in recovery) member, always the youngest. But Father Time
takes care of that small dilemma by allowing us to
accumulate many single days in the Program that add
up to months and years.

I'm no longer the most important person in
the meetings. Instead, I'm just a very grateful member.

82.   LIVE A LITTLE -- JUST TO PLEASE

Can you say today in honesty
As the hours slip by so fast,
That you've helped a single person
Of the many you have passed?

Did you waste the day, or lose it?
Was it well, properly spent?
Did you leave a trail of kindness
Or mementos of discontent?

Have you given God a moment
In humble, devout prayer?
Have you talked with Him in honesty
To let Him know you care?

As you close your eyes in slumber,
Do you think that God would say,
"You have made the world much better,
For you *lived a lot* today"?

83.   HOW THE SLOGANS HELPED ME

When I first heard that "we get sober on the
SLOGANS and stay sober on the TWELVE STEPS, I
hardly knew what the slogans were. After I learned
about them, I wondered if "my way" wasn't just the
opposite. Although I try to live the Twelve Steps each
day, the slogans have been a very important part of my
recovery. The slogans give me hope and courage when
I'm frightened and worried.

I was in the hospital with a back problem after
shoveling snow. Obviously, my bad back was the result
of my activity, and yet, I did wonder. The reason for my
questioning was because a friend, who had been hos-
pitalized with a bad back, had recently been diagnosed
as having cancer.

Although I was praying, reading my books and talking to fellow members and family, I couldn't seem to "Let Go." Finally, the slogans came to my rescue as I was able to combine them in a kind of prayer. It was "This too will pass" if I "Let Go and Let God" "One day at a time" and "Accept the things I cannot change!" That still helps me when I get in a tight spot.

84.   RELAPSE OVER GUILT

Though I know how hurt and sorry you must be after your relapse, please do not worry about a temporary loss of your inner peace. As calmly as you can, just renew your effort on the Program, especially those parts of it which have to do with meditation and self-analysis.

Could I also suggest that you look at excessive guilt for what it is, nothing but a sort of reverse pride? A decent regret for what has happened is fine, but guilt? No.

Indeed, the relapse could well have been brought about by unreasonable feelings of guilt because of other moral failures, so called. Surely, you ought to look into this possibility. Even here you should not blame yourself for failure; you can be penalized only for refusing to try for better things.

85.   FOUR PARADOXES OF THE PROGRAM

1.   You have to get sick to get well.
2.   You have to surrender to win.
3.   You have to die to be born again.
4.   You have to give it away to keep it.

86.   MIDDLE AGE SPREAD
(Activity vs. complacency)

Did you know there's a "Middle Age Spread" for the average 12-Step member? It's that time when you're not new anymore and you don't have the wisdom of the old-timer yet. You find yourself somewhere in the middle, being "spread" pretty thin, doing far more than you think you should, but you're not sure. You're sponsoring several new people, going to a couple of extra meetings a week, and the phone is ringing off the wall. Ah! This is the life! Or is it? Is this really what the Program suggests? What has happened to moderation, Easy Does It, Live and Let Live, and But For the Grace of God?

Stop a moment and think about or visualize this person, and you see one busy member, spreading themselves too thin. I have a sneaking suspicion that people pleasing and needing acceptance are at the bottom of this problem, plus a pinch of restlessness.

The ailment can be arrested, much like the physical "middle age spread," by going on a diet, using some God and self power. Ask Him for the willingness to accept the truth, to recognize it when it comes. Use the discipline to say yes or no when you should try to abstain from the needless running around.

It's not easy for me to stop the "middle age spread." It's so subtle and I lack self-discipline. But to admit a need for help and to have a willingness to try is half the battle. How about you who are suffering from the "middle age spread"? *Complacency*, on the other hand, is the opposite half of this dilemma. Complacency is that condition which settles in when indifference to growth has entered one's life. It is equally disruptive and destructive. With complacency there is a feeling of no need to move at all, a false feeling that all is well. How deceiving this subtle foe is.

The middle of the road is our goal. Let's journey together, greeting one another as we each return periodically from our side trips down the wrong road. Character is the Tree, Reputation is the Shadow, Recovery is our Friend. God's light forever shines upon those who are willing to step out into it.

87.   LOVING OURSELVES
(Low self-esteem)

We often hear that we must love ourselves, and we wonder how this is done. We're told, "take care of yourself," "pat yourself on the back," or "look in the mirror and tell yourself, 'I love you'." We try these things and still find ourselves rejecting ourselves.

That's where some of us were; that's where some of us are. Low self-esteem has to be one of the greatest dilemmas facing us in 12-Step recovery. But aren't we fortunate, in the Program, to have the tools with which to help build and maintain self-esteem, self-love, and self-acceptance?

These helpful tools are the *action* Steps (4 through 9) of the 12-Step Program. Possibly the most important thing we learn in working these Steps is how to accept and forgive others and ourselves. As we list our resentments and analyze them, sometimes we see where we were wrong; sometimes we don't. It is of little importance who is right or who is wrong, only that we accept and forgive. And if we are willing to work this Program and have forgiveness for others, then we begin and become willing to forgive ourselves.

For if we continue to feel anger, guilt, shame, and remorse, these self-resentments will block us from the "Sunshine of the Spirit" just as surely as any resentment against another person will. We will be forever stuck at the side of the road, not proceeding with our fellow travelers down the road of recovery.

And if we're stuck, we'd better take another look at the God of our understanding. In Chapter Four of the Big Book ("We Agnostics"), it says: *"We found the Great Reality deep down within us. In the last analysis it is only there that He may be found. It was so with us."*

By not accepting and forgiving ourselves for the wrongs of yesterday, whether it be the recent yesterday or the yesterday of yore, we cannot find the "Great Reality" within us. It is only when we get rid of the garbage of self-hate and negative self-talk that we find and love God and ourselves.

88.   NOT A SINGLES' BAR OR A LONELY HEARTS' CLUB
(Step 13)

I often hear it said that there's a shortage of women in the Program who are willing and able to sponsor other women. I don't know how true that is; but I do know that, as a long-time female member, I am approached very often with a request to sponsor some fairly new person, or with a request to share a Fifth Step with them. I never refuse, and by the grace of God so far I have had the strength and, hopefully, the wisdom, to be of some help. I am certainly willing to *try*.

Out of these many talks with young and not so young, new and not so new, female members, one very negative and damaging trend stands out above all the other pitfalls on the road to recovery, and that is the problem of "wolves in sheep's clothing" who prowl some of our meetings. Countless young women have had unwelcome advances forced on them when as little as one week in the Program, and in two cases I know of girls who were approached at their first meeting and were so disgusted that they never returned. If these "wolves" were relative newcomers themselves, there would perhaps be some excuse; but most of them are of several years' duration in the Program, abstinent maybe, but certainly not living the principles.

Consider the words of A.A.'s Step 12: "Having had a spiritual awakening as the result of these steps, we tried to carry *this message* to alcoholics and practice *these principles* in all our affairs." What is *this message*? Surely it is one of discipline and self-control in our own lives, coupled with a loving concern and desire to help our fellow members. Certainly it has nothing to do with a selfish lust, no matter what flowery phrase may be used to disguise it. What are *these principles* we try to practice in all our affairs? The literature tells us that the principles behind the Program are those of Honesty, Purity, Unselfishness and

Love, and try as I might, I cannot turn that around to read, "Satisfy No. 1 at all costs, no matter who gets hurt in the process." Strong stuff, I know, but I feel it's time it was said. Yes, I know we're all supposed to take our own inventories, and "Live and Let Live," but when girls and women coming into the Program are at risk of being put off a live-saving Program by these hustlers out for their own selfish gratification, and when they are too new and unsure to stand up for themselves, it's time to bring this exploitation out into the open.

Having said all that, there are countless good men in the Program; and I have received great help and good advice from them, for which I am very grateful. I enjoy male company immensely, and some of my closest friends are of the opposite sex, so please don't get the idea I'm a man-hater or a radical feminist; it's simply a question that "if the cap fits, wear it." If not, disregard it. And please, please, all you good members out there, male and female, if you too become aware of trends or continuous occurrences which may be in danger of eroding the fabric or good name of our Program, *do* have the courage of your convictions and speak up about it. It's not always the case that "Silence Is Golden."

We owe it to those still suffering to come and stand up and be counted and not to allow a small percentage of misguided members to destroy a Fellowship which, to my mind, has no equal. No one member represents our Fellowship, but *every member* has a responsibility to guard its good name. For that, we are all responsible.

89.   PROCRASTINATION
(Steps 4 and 11)

"I'll do it tomorrow" is a habit that leaves you always behind schedule. If yesterday's work is only getting done today, then how can today's work get done? It has, of course, to wait until tomorrow. Can you catch up? No. You are in the habit of procrastinating. You have a black cloud over your head, made up of guilt, anxiety, worry. A feeling of failure creeps in.

In the Program it's "A Day At A Time." We try to do today's work today. What if we put off the first step of the work? No job, even school, office, or career will give us satisfaction unless we see the value of our day's work. Satisfaction comes from doing the job on time, reaching our goal "just for today." If procrastination had an effect on only oneself, it wouldn't be so bad. But no, it puts a strain on those around us. Tight schedules leave little time for conversation or for relaxed meal times, and no time to fit into the family activities. Procrastination tends to lock you out of your community, even the community of the Program. For how can you share when you are in a state of mind which is preoccupied with yourself and your problems?

Working on this character defect will allow you to participate in your personal and Fellowship life. The ability to concentrate, to use your time well, is everything. It is self-control. It's the Program in action. The Fourth Step speaks of instinct gone wild. We must get control of our instincts. When you are tired you have feelings of uneasiness. These feelings come from stress, the strain of always rushing around. But the feeling of uneasiness also comes from an undernourished spirit, a spirit that never has time to go away to a quiet place and rest awhile. The Eleventh Step seeks the will of God. Have we not enough in today's own troubles without making a double load for tomorrow?

Benjamin Franklin said, *"Do you love life? Then do not squander time, for that is the stuff life is made of."* The Twelve Steps are the same for everyone. We are all given the choice, the means to break the habit of procrastination, so we may be free to strive for spiritual growth in our lives.

90.   LISTENING?

How often have you wanted to be heard by your family or friends? The times you couldn't say what was wrong, but prayed someone else might just pick up on the problem? When I was drinking, I was a master at this. I wanted *them* to see how bad I was suffering, and if they didn't, out came the bottle. *Because* no one understood me. I never listened either. I rattled on like a guitar in the hands of a child. "Nothing made sense," I said.

The day the Master picked me up, and I began practicing the A.A. principles in all my affairs, is the day I got in tune with you. Listening gets answers we need. Listening gives support others need. Advice is cheap if it doesn't flow through us from God. Do you ever get in the way and block off an answer? I do.

Some day, just sit alone among the trees, listening. The birds are an orchestra. Listen to the laughter of a child playing. A rabbit came almost up to me this morning. It brought tears to my eyes. Why? Because a few light years ago my family stayed out of a rock's throw of me. Now animals are comfortable around me because I'm comfortable with me. Give me a good listener any day with a Big Book and enough time, and I'll come up with His answer.

91.   MY BILL OF RIGHTS

I have the right to:
be treated with respect.
say no and not feel guilty.

experience and express my feelings.

take time for myself.

change my mind.

ask for what I want.

ask for information.

make mistakes.

do less than I am humanly capable of.

feel good about myself.

act only in ways that promote my dignity and self-respect as long as others' are not violated in the process.

92.   PRAYER IS A SPECIAL TIME

Prayer is a special time I share with God. Prayer is the means I use to talk with God and to listen as God communicates with me. When I pray, I become still and quiet any unrest within me. I reaffirm my oneness with my Higher Power and I find the answers I seek.

I do not limit my prayers to a certain time or a particular place. Whenever a small success enters my life or a moment of joy illumines my day, I silently thank God for those blessings. Every time I affirm God as the source of my good and give thanks for the many channels through which it comes, I am praying to God.

Prayer enables me to know and to feel that I

am a beloved child of God. I am needed because I can be an expression of good in my world.

93.   IN OUR ACCEPTANCE LIES OUR SOLUTION

In being able to accept the things we did, the thoughts we have, and the feelings we have, finally comes the peace I so long for. Even a few people can love me today; and my past bad behavior, thoughts and feelings become a positive, creative part of my life.

For a while the solution seems more like a paradox because I find myself having to accept the things I don't like. It is interesting to discover in doing this kind of evaluation I can finally get to something better. It seems there is never any value in going around the problems or pushing down the feeling; rather, taking a look and accepting the truth helps me set up my own rules in life and helps me find out what really makes me feel better about who and what I am.

When I first came in, I couldn't wait until I could get it all together. Then as time went by, I realized I probably never would get it all together and really maybe I shouldn't try. Trying to get it all together keeps me from surrender. I discovered in surrendering everything to my Higher Power I was given more feelings of peace in my life.

Why is it always so easy to complicate everything? Oh well, that's how I learn! Members used to tell me it's because you're an addict; just accept it! So much of what they taught me was so simple, and through this simple way, I learned to surrender all and peace takes over my life again.

94.   GRATITUDE FOR SPIRITUALITY

Before I came to the Program I knew of a God. I didn't know Him personally and didn't care to know Him either. Evolution and the science aspect of our creation was what I believed in. My idea of God was that if I were to bare my soul to Him I would be condemned and be struck by lightning. I realize now that that was an excuse not to "Let Go and Let God" for me. I was terrified of working a Third Step. I was terrified of surrender also. I asked myself, "If I let go will God take care of me? Will God not fail me?" That, for me, was lack of faith.

Today, I have surrendered, and I work my Third Step to the best of my ability. Today, I have "come to believe in a Power greater than myself." I have "made the decision to turn it over to a Power greater than myself."

For me this has been a real turning point. I no longer have to fight. I don't have nearly as much fear as I did, because my Higher Power is always with me.

Today my Higher Power takes care of me and He makes choices, I don't. If I can't handle a person, place, or thing, I turn it over. I can't do it all by myself. My Higher Power does it for me.

95.   ARE YOU WILLING

Are you willing:

To forget what you have done for other people and to remember what other people have done for you.

To ignore what the world owes you and to think what you owe the world.

To put your rights in the background and your duties in the middle distance and your chances to do a little more than your duty in the foreground.

To see that other people are just as real as you are and try to look behind their faces to their hearts, hungry for joy as you are.

To own that probably the only good reason for your existence is not what you are going to to get out of life but what you are going to give to life.

To close your book of complaints against the management of the universe and look for a place where you can sow a few seeds of happiness.

Are you willing to do these things even for a day? Then you have a good chance of continuing your recovery.

96.   STAYING IN TOUCH
(Back to Step 1)

I've noticed that something happens to some of us after the first few years in recovery. We become dissatisfied. We begin to find fault with the meetings and the people at them. We want more.

We find other things to do with our time. After all, it's been some time since we had to think about using, and we reason that we don't need meetings to stay abstinent.

Besides, after all our hard work, we deserve a break. With all this time in the Program, isn't it time to be normal?

This line of reasoning should flash DANGER, but we have a disease that tells us we're not that sick.

It is surely right and good that we should get to the point that we want to do more than just go to meetings. I believe that our Higher Power has helped us so we can become useful, active members of society. But left to myself and my disease-thinking, I will soon believe that my answers are "out there."

No matter how many 24 hours I've been abstinent, I need to come back to hear the message that my answers come through working the Twelve Steps.

An important point I think we sometimes forget is that we owe our lives to the Program. The grace of God through the Fellowship has blessed me with the options to live and to join the human race. I can begin to give back a little of what was given to me by doing my share to make sure the meetings are there for the next newcomer. By passing on what was given to me, others can have the option to live.

If I'm not at the meeting that process can't occur, and then, I believe, we are all at risk. Let's not cheat ourselves and the Fellowship in pursuit of some delusion we call a "normal" life. We have a disease that progresses even as we recover, so I doubt we can ever truly be "normal."

If we're having trouble accepting that, then it's back to Step One and more meetings. Isn't that what we'd tell the newcomer?

97.   ENDINGS VS. BEGINNINGS

I rarely could look at any of life's experiences as an opportunity for a new beginning. I always concentrated on the ending and hated for it to happen, whether it was good or bad. I hung onto relationships that should have ended, worked at jobs too long, and refused to give up on "old ideas" (still do some of the time).

Even when I started something new, I projected the end; and it was never going to be good.

The Program tells me that I must close a door so that a new door will open. But I hesitate doing so, because I want to know what's behind the new door before risking it.

Whenever something ended, it seemed like the end of the world to me. I am slowly becoming aware that it "ain't necessarily so."

It's a relief to find out that I can fail at something and that doesn't have to be the end. I can start all over, make a new beginning. I ordinarily wouldn't even start if I thought I was doomed to fail. Today, I try not to project "the end" and work at whatever I am doing just for today.

Endings don't frighten me today like they used to, because I am starting to realize for every ending there will be a new beginning.

98.   NO REGRETS

Isn't it good at the end of the day
To look up to God and be able to say
"Dear Lord, I helped someone today."
But isn't it sad if instead you must say
"Dear Lord, I hurt someone today.
I drove the nails a little bit deeper
And forgot that I am my brother's keeper."

Isn't it better when the day is done
To know that you have injured no one.
From the time of your waking,
Till you lie down to sleep,
Remember the promises that we should keep.
To love one another as He loves us too,
And you'll never regret any good that you do.

99.   MY SPONSOR

I don't remember reading anything in the Big Book that says you've gotta have a sponsor, but I don't think I could have ever gotten sober without mine, and I don't see how anyone else could.

I've heard a lot of people say in meetings that alcohol made them sweetly reasonable. It never did that for me. It made me mean and crazy and unreasonable and sick. It was my sponsor who made me reasonable. By sharing her experience, strength and hope with me, she convinced me I had a choice as to whether I would drink or not drink. That was big news to me! She sent me to A.A.!

But even after becoming reasonable enough to choose not to drink, it took nearly a year of A.A. and her patience and tolerance and guidance before I had what I like to call the "spiritual experience" that enabled me to quit. It was after this experience that she told me I was finally, FINALLY, teachable!!! We started with Step One for the umpteenth time and proceeded from there.

Together we built a foundation for a new way of life. The materials we used came from the Program of Alcoholics Anonymous, the Twelve Steps, the meetings, the people, the service work. The master planner was a Higher Power whom I came to know as a loving God that I could trust to do what's best for me.

She showed me how to integrate the principles and concepts of the A.A. Program into a way of living that continues to expand and develop as I do. It makes the process of growing up tolerable, something I'd never been able to do.

One of the greatest gifts my sponsor gave me is the knowledge that she did not get me sober. She's told me that not only my sobriety, but everything else I expect to get out of my life, is contingent upon my conscious, continuous contact with a Power greater than her and me and everyone else all put together; and this is the knowledge I try to pass on to those I sponsor.

100. LEARNING TO BE A FRIEND

I never realized how difficult it is to be a friend. For years I tried to control every relationship I was in, and I smothered anyone I called friend. It has been hard to let go of that tendency.

I always had only one friend at a time, and I thought that person had to be my friend exclusively. To be called "one of my friends" by someone to whom I gave all my attention felt like a slight to me. After all, this person was *my* only friend, and I wanted sole rights to her friendship.

Thanks to two years in the Program I can see my errors. My exclusivity brought isolation. If my one and only friend wasn't available, I was alone. Now I have a network of beautiful, loving friends. As I reach out, I find that contact with others brings a new dimension to old relationships. I learn something from each person, and I become a better friend.

Still, I am sometimes apt to confuse love with smothering and stifling. There's the old urge to control people by "saving" them. If someone hurts, I have a band-aid; for every bad time, I have a solution.

It takes a great deal of Program not to try to run everyone's life, but I'm working at it. Daily, I ask God's help in releasing my friends to the care of their Higher Power.

A true friend listens without judging, helps without solving, loves without clinging. A friend has a number of interests and engages in a variety of activities that serve to enliven a friendship. A friend is there when needed, but respects the other's need for privacy.

There is something almost mythically idealistic about this portrait of a friend. I may never reach that ideal, but I am trying my best, and that's all I can do. This Program calls for progress, not perfection.

101. IF I HAD MY LIFE TO LIVE OVER

I'd like to make more mistakes next time. I'd relax. I would limber up. I would be sillier than I have been this trip. I would take fewer things seriously. I would take more chances. I would climb more mountains and swim more rivers. I would eat more ice cream and fewer beans. I would perhaps have more actual troubles, but I'd have fewer imaginary ones.

You see, I'm one of those people who live sensibly and sanely hour after hour, day after day. Oh, I've had my moments, and if I had it to do over again, I'd have more of them. In fact, I'd try to have nothing else; just moments, one after another, instead of living so many years ahead of each day. I've been one of those persons who never goes anywhere without a thermometer, a hot water bottle, a raincoat, and a parachute. If I had to do it again, I would travel lighter than I have.

If I had my life to live over, I would start barefoot earlier in the spring and stay that way later in the fall. I would go to more dances. I would ride more merry-go-rounds. I would pick more daisies.

102.   SOMEONE TO TRUST
(Step 5)

Something I heard recently keeps running through my mind. "What Step were you working when you relapsed?" I haven't relapsed, that is I haven't picked up, but I'm not working a Step. I'm sitting on the Fifth Step. It's a rather uncomfortable place to sit.

The Fifth Step is where you admit to God, yourself, and another human being the exact nature of your wrongs. The only part that bothers me about the Fifth Step is the "another human being" part. I'm not a trusting soul. I know God is working in my life. I see the evidence of His presence in every single day of my life. But God, to tell someone EVERYTHING. Can't we keep this just between us?

I'm in recovery today, and for someone like me that is a miracle. But to stay, I must do the Steps as they are written. I must learn to trust that God will put that someone special in my path and the courage will come.

That special someone is usually a sponsor. My sponsor moved away a year ago, and I just haven't felt like trusting anyone again. Sponsorship is a very special privilege. To help someone through the Steps by sharing your experience, strength and hope must be very fulfilling. It's an honor I hope to have someday, when my own house is in order.

My only advice to anyone getting ready to take a Fifth would be: TAKE IT BEFORE THE INK IS DRY so your EGO can't get in the way.

103.   I SAID A PRAYER FOR YOU TODAY

I said a prayer for you today
And know God must have heard.
I felt the answer in my heart
Although God spoke no word.
I didn't ask for wealth or fame
(I knew you wouldn't mind).
I asked God to send treasures
Of a far more lasting kind.
I asked that God would be near you
At the start of each new day
To grant you health and blessings
And friends to share your way.
I asked for happiness for you
In all things great and small,
But it was for God's loving care
I prayed the most of all.

104.   WHAT A GREAT FRIEND

What a great friend you are to me!
What a great person to give love so free!
You've helped me a lot, just to watch me smile,
Let me know that you care and life is worthwhile.

Change doesn't come easy, I'm the first to agree,
But taking it slowly really works for me.
I don't know about tomorrow; I only know today.
I won't live life in sorrow; I'm going a new way.
I'll never be perfect, like I once thought I would.
But I'll be the best I can, and that's pretty good!

You've helped me be stronger than ever before,
Made me believe in myself; I can't ask for more.
What a great friend you are to me!
What a great person to give love so free!

105.   THIS, TOO, SHALL PASS
   (When?)

The pain is worse than you can ever remember. You look up and say the Serenity Prayer and nothing happens. You pace the floor and then sit down, and then get up and fix another cup of coffee, and then take a deep breath and wait.

"This, too, shall pass" is like a scratched record in your brain, and you wonder: When? And you don't relapse.

You drive and turn the radio up loud to drown out the thoughts, then stop to look over the city from the hill. You cry, and you hurt.

Each day after each sleepless night, you ask, "Is this the day, God? Is this the day when it will be over?" And each day, it isn't.

You stay in when it rains. You stay in when the sun shines. You don't notice the difference. Food doesn't go down. You go to meetings.

You cover up, and you smile and ache. You call a friend, and it doesn't help. You feel as if you will explode if you don't unload on someone, and then you finally do. It brings a little relief. And you keep working the Program.

You say the Serenity Prayer ten times with closed eyes and clenched fists. You beat the pillow with your fists, look at the clock, and know you have made it through one more day, one minute at a time. You hurt some more.

Then the day comes. You open the door, and the sun is shining and warm. You see the trees. And you say, "Is this the day, God?" And it is.

106.   NEVER HAD A CHANCE

Yes, I'm an alcoholic, addict, overeater--you name it. I also grew up in an abusive alcoholic home. I've been in recovery now for four years, clean and sober and being consistent in eating the right foods.

Some information I received early on in recovery has been a help to me. Because of some genetic or other imbalance in my brain, I guess I never had a chance at being "normal." One can read extensively on this subject (most commonly called the "X Factor") or talk to experts, but they're a long way from finding the exact factors in the brain that make some of us susceptible to addiction.

This knowledge helped me get out of the shame and stop blaming myself for all the negative events in my life. I do remind myself that I have responsibility for some of the things that went on. Gradually, in early recovery, I began to accept my disease, and became willing to do my best to live a different life; basically, I learned to know the difference between what's right or wrong, good or bad for me.

Perhaps I never had a chance to be "normal," but the Program and other help available has given me an opportunity to be a better me. I know I am less depressed when I eat right, lay off the sugar, and get a little exercise. I've learned to trust again; first the

Program, then other people. The Eighth and Ninth
Steps have helped me forgive my father for his abuse.
        It's been very hard work at times, but the
Steps and my fellow members have pulled me through.
This *is* a better way to live.

107.   SIGNS OF A SPIRITUAL
          AWAKENING

A tendency to think and act spontaneously rather than
on fears based on past experiences.
An unmistakable ability to enjoy each moment.
A loss of interest in judging people.
A loss of interest in judging self.
A loss of interest in interpreting the actions of others.
A loss of interest in conflict.
A loss of ability to worry. (This is a serious symptom.)
Frequent, overwhelming episodes of appreciation.
Contented feelings of connectedness with others and
nature.
Frequent attacks of smiling.
An increased tendency to let things happen rather than
make them happen.
An increased susceptibility to the love extended by
others as well as the uncontrollable urge to extend it.

108.   A NEW OUTLOOK
(Al-Anon)

Facing reality and accepting responsibility for my own actions were the most difficult challenges for me to face when sobriety became a reality in my home. Up to that point, anger, resentment, and denial blinded me to the fact that I was allowing another person to control my actions. I was avoiding responsibility for my own actions.

Reality was frightening. The old saying, "what you don't know won't hurt you," doesn't apply to people affected by alcoholism. What I didn't know was what kept me in a sick situation. What I couldn't see was that I was *re*-acting instead of acting. The biggest problem at that point was knowing how to act.

Al-Anon saved me! After the first few meetings I realized that no one would outline my life for me. Rather, there were guidelines that I was free to follow; tools that were at my disposal. I needed fellowship, understanding, support; Al-Anon gave that to me. At meetings I learned that no one could make me completely happy or completely unhappy. Through practicing the Steps, new habits became part of my life, habits that lead to healthy relationships and a new outlook on life. Thank you, Al-Anon friends, for caring enough to share!

109. WISDOM

Wisdom is not necessarily the ability to recite
the 12 Steps in their correct order, say all the slogans,
remember lots of quotations from the literature. It's
just being ourselves, working the Program as we see it
and having continued faith in our Higher Power.
Wisdom is God-given. It has little to do with reading
all the pamphlets and books and believing that's all
that is known. Just read them again in six months' time
and wonder who published the new books!

I have met many old-timers and have found
that in almost all cases they have an inner peace not so
evident in many of us. They have grasped the real
meaning of EASY DOES IT. They seldom rush in and
become involved in side issues but tend to think things
out first.

Now don't get me wrong. I don't mean they
are right more often than us, but with God on their side
they tend to lose a little less. The important things are
really important to them.

Wisdom has little to do with our mental
ability. With our Higher Power alongside us, we can
achieve anything, even long-term recovery ONE DAY
AT A TIME. In our Serenity Prayer, we ask God for
wisdom and patience. It will come, as a result of
treating our Program, the meetings, and the message
as precious things that really matter. Wisdom comes

to ordinary people like ourselves who try to live the program ONE DAY AT A TIME, not overnight, but as the accumulation of many 24 hours. Wisdom comes with practice, the practice of living a new way of life, a spiritual life resulting from our 12 Step Program.

110.   GOD'S GIFT OF LOVE

God's love is like an island
In life's ocean vast and wide,
A peaceful, quiet shelter
From the restless, rising tide.
God's love is like a fortress
And we seek protection there,
When the waves of tribulation
Seem to drown us in despair.
God's love is like a beacon
Burning bright with faith and prayer;
And through the changing scenes of life,
We can find a Haven there.

111.   LOVE IS NOT--

Love is not something we can search for and find, except within ourselves.
Love is not something that just happens; it takes work and patience and effort.

We spend so much time looking for the right person to love or finding fault with those we already love, when instead we should be perfecting the love we give to others.

This is the only way we can ever truly be satisfied with anyone or anything; for in loving, we find love itself.

112.   LOVE IS--

Love is patient; love is kind and is not jealous; love does not brag and is not arrogant.

Love does not act unbecomingly; it does not seek its own, is not provoked, does not take into account a wrong suffered.

Love does not rejoice in unrighteousness, but rejoices in the truth.

Love bears all things, believes all things, endures all things.

Love never fails.

113.   WHY SMILE?

It's not easy to smile when you feel the world is kicking you in the teeth and everything you touch seems to turn into ashes. But you can do it, if you try.

Think about it for a moment and you'll realize that you know some individual who has shown that it can be done, someone who has had more than one person's share of disappointments and setbacks and yet manages to walk with head high and with an outward smile to the world.

Why smile? Why pretend that life is a bed of roses when it's nothing more than a bag of thorns? Simply because a smile is an outward sign of an inner determination to persist, to carry on.

Anyone can quit. Some do it by rolling over and playing dead. Others quit by walking away, believing foolishly that troubles will not follow.

Keep your smile and never lose it. A smile is a sign of strength and confidence. A smile is a sign of faith strong enough to hang in there and keep trying until something can be done about troubles and problems. A smile is recognition of the fact that troubles are nothing more than temporary inconveniences along the road of life.

114. AS YOU THINK--

As you think, you travel; and as you love, you attract. You are today where your thoughts have brought you; you will be tomorrow where your thoughts take you. You cannot escape the result of your thoughts; but you can endure and learn, can accept and be glad. You will realize the vision (not the idle wish) of your

heart, be it base or beautiful, or a mixture of both, for
you will always gravitate toward that which you secretly most love. Into your hands will be placed the
exact result of your thoughts; you will receive that
which you earn, no more, no less. Whatever your
present environment may be, you will fall, remain, or
rise with your thoughts, your vision, your ideal. You
will become as small as your controlling desire, as
great as your dominant aspiration.

115. SMALL CONTRIBUTIONS, BIG GROWTH
(Step 12)

Someone in the Program told me early on
that we teach what we most want to learn. By sharing
our experience, strength, and hope with others, we
somehow come to learn the things which we are most
hungry to learn. I have experienced the reality of this
concept many, many times. It is always true that when
I work with others, I receive the healing for which I was
either consciously or unconsciously looking.

I remember how reluctant I was at first to
work with others or to do service work. You see, I was
far too busy and in entirely too much pain to have to
hassle with some newcomer who was babbling nonsense and being hysterical. No, no, no. What I was

going to do was get my act together first and then save
the whole lot in one fell swoop and go serenely about
my very important life. Well, let me tell ya, sweetheart,
that ain't the way it works!

Fortunately, I have been maneuvered into
sharing by some pretty crafty veteran members. By
simply massaging my ego, they managed to get me
involved in sponsorship, speaking at meetings, etc.,
and what happened is truly a miracle. My small
contributions have been rewarded with personal growth
beyond compare.

Every time I work with someone new, I learn
more about the Program and more about myself. It's
as if the bitter pill I thought service work would be
turned out to be the sweetest cure for what ails me.
The point of all this being: give yourself a gift, by
giving. It will be the nicest thing you ever did for you.

116.   I AM ADDICTION

I am more powerful than the combined armies of the
world.
I have destroyed more people than all the wars of the
nation.
I have caused millions of accidents and wrecked more
homes than all the floods, tornadoes and hurricanes
put together.

I am the world's slickest thief.

I steal billions of dollars each year.

I find my victims among the rich and poor alike, the young and the old, the strong and the weak.

I loom up to such proportions that I cast a shadow over every field of labor.

I am relentless, insidious, unpredictable;

I am everywhere: in the home, on the street, in the factory, in the office, on the sea and in the air.

I bring sickness, poverty and death.

I give nothing and take all.

I am your worst enemy.

I am addiction.

117. WHAT DID YOU DO TODAY?

So you've been around for many years. You worked like hell when you first came in, but what did you do today?

I heard your pitch, it was kind of long; you really told them how. You worked the Steps in '71, but how are you working them now?

Do you still get up from your soft warm bed when someone is in trouble?

Or have you forgotten the early times when you were sort of new? Maybe you've been around so long that the Program is old hat to you?

Maybe you're one of the Senior Saints, serene and satisfied; and you've forgotten when you were sick and when you damn near died?

Maybe I shouldn't bring it up; maybe you're too blase'. But just for the hell of it, what did you do today?

Have you been around so cockeyed long you leave it to Mary and Sam, because you're not your brother's keeper and don't give a damn?

Maybe tonight a good T.V. show is on, or you're going to the movies. So what the hell if a person is sick; they have only themselves to blame.

Well, you have a perfect right to work your own Program; and you know you'll do it your own way no matter what I say. But tonight before you go to bed, just look in the glass and pray that you and the Lord know the answer to WHAT DID YOU DO TODAY?

118. THE LANGUAGE OF THE HEART

For thirty years I lived in my head and spoke the language generated from what I saw as my most powerful tool, my brain. I relied on that power and basked in the glory of its accomplishments. I had notions that the language of my heart, specifically my feelings, must be kept out of the way and concealed in order to allow my head to be in control. The roadblock I constructed between my heart and my head caused me much pain and frustration; there was a void in my life that only my addiction could fill. That power to numb pain became my highest power until the day I realized it had taken control of my life.

It is in the Fellowship that I have had the awesome experience of traveling from my head to my heart and learned to speak the language of the heart. It is in these rooms I discovered that God resided in my heart; and it was there I found love, joy, laughter, along with the realities of pain and sorrow I had hidden from for so long. The language of my heart uses fewer words; it feels more than it speaks; it listens more than it preaches; it touches the hearts of others without a single word; it is only comfortable with the truth. It is through this language that I feel alive today; I am a participant in life rather than an observer. I speak to my fellows and my God with the language of my heart, and am most grateful to have been given this second chance.

119. FATAL MISTAKES

A person struck a match to see if the gasoline tank in their car was empty. It wasn't!

A person patted a strange dog on the head to

see if the dog was affectionate. It wasn't!

A person sped up to see if they could beat the train to the crossing. They couldn't!

A person touched an electrical wire to see if the power was off. It wasn't!

A member went back out after a long period of recovery to see if they could control it again and do it their way instead of the 12-Step way. They couldn't!

120.   I'VE FOUND ME

The love of God
I've found within.
It's the greatest gift,
To begin again.
New meanings,
New choices,
New horizons,
New ways to be,
I've found them all,
Because I've found me.

121.   KINDNESS

The greatest lever to move the hearts of people is by acts of kindness. Kindness is the prime factor in overcoming friction and in making human machinery run more smoothly.

If a man or woman, mistakenly, is your enemy, you cannot disarm them so surely in any other way as by doing them a kindly act.

Yes, if we are strong enough to do a kindness to someone who has wronged us, there is no more certain way of bringing about restitution than by an act of sincere kindness, either by word of mouth or by hand.

As Shakespeare would have said it, "It is twice blessed; it blesses her that gives and she that receives." Further, the person who can overcome their frailties and prejudices toward another person who may have wronged them increases their own moral and spiritual strength, by rising above themselves!

Kindness is one thing that you cannot give away. It always comes back!

122. RECOVERY--A TIME FOR LEARNING

"When the pupil is ready, the teacher appears." Life's lessons often come unexpectedly. They come, nevertheless; and they come according to a time frame that is set by our Higher Power. As we grow emotionally and spiritually, we are readied for further lessons for which teachers will appear.

Perhaps the teacher will be a tragic experience, a loving relationship, or a difficult loss. The time of learning is seldom free from pain and questioning, but from these experiences and what they can teach us, we are ready to learn. As we are ready, they come.

For life has much to teach us, just as we have much to learn. We need to learn patience, for the learning and growing process is usually slow. We need to learn tolerance, for we are being taught that it is more important to understand than to be understood. We need to learn self-respect, for only when we have learned to love ourselves better can we love others better.

We are learning that there is a right time for all growth, a right time for all experience; and the right time may not fit our timetable. What does not come our way today will come when the time is right. Each day we are granted just what is needed. We need not worry about the future. It will offer us whatever rightly comes next, but it cannot do so until we have experienced those 24 hours before us.

123.   TRY ACCEPTANCE!

A problem is a set of circumstances that threatens your well-being. And what are "circumstances"? Circumstances are people and things. So "solving our problems" really means getting people and things the way we want them. Sometimes we can do it. More often we can't. What then?

There are several things we can do. We can look around to find somebody or something to blame. Or we can put ashes in our hair, wear shabby shoes with rundown heels, accentuate our wrinkles, and make the rounds of our friends chanting, "Poor me, poor me!" We can succeed in making our family miserable. We can haunt doctors. We can waylay our sponsor, beat our breast, and blame God with, "What have I done to deserve this?"

If you are desperate enough, you will try anything. So try something that works: try acceptance! It can be acquired if you have an urgent desire to help yourself and are willing to ask God to help you.

124.   SERVICE KEEPS IT WORKING

One day the radio antenna on my car refused to work. It was pointed out that I had neglected to service it, a small matter of wiping it clean occasionally.

My car antenna does not work unless I service it. My Program does not work unless I service it. The whole Program of meetings, fellowship, and sponsorship depends upon the service of individual members.

At first we serve because we are told. As the

days pass we begin to offer service, each in our own way, out of genuine caring for the people and the Program.

The rewards? Because we have a tendency to be self-centered, the unfailing byproduct is forgetting for the moment that which causes us most, if not all, of our troubles: ourselves.

Many a troubled day is smoothed by an act, if only a prayer of service.

125.   LIFE IS TOO SHORT TO BE LITTLE

This is a world filled with trouble for all of us. It doesn't matter who we are, how highly educated or uneducated we may be; we all see both bright and dark mental pictures.

Many people go through life wearing smoked mental glasses. They never realize there are many happy hours to be enjoyed if they could change their thinking. They cause unhappiness for themselves because they cannot make others act or think the way they believe they should.

At times I feel disgusted, not only with myself, because of the way I sometimes think and act, but with the way other people think and act.

If we were wise enough to realize how little we

know and stop trying to make others think we have
more of what it takes to get along in this world than we
really have, it would help us.

"The top" is never reached. When we feel we
"have arrived" we soon learn we have just begun; and
the more we depend upon ourselves to reach our
objective the steeper the hills and the more crooked
the road we are traveling becomes.

How little we really are and how difficult it is
for many of us to realize our weakness. Of course,
many of us do, but we still put on the same old "phony
front" and seem to enjoy making ourselves unhappy by
trying to make a good impression. Many men and
women who spread manure around the farmyard barn
lot when young saturate themselves with rank perfume
because the manufacturer claims it is the "daintiest of
daintiest!" odor. Of course, they cannot be blamed.
After years of cow manure all over one's clothes,
perhaps a change of smell really does some people
good.

Man has found a formula for almost everything learned men and women have discovered, but
nobody has discovered a way to carry on alone. We
must have, and do receive, "outside" help. If not, we
will stumble and fall and eventually be unable to rise.

Every morning before I start out to do "battle"
with life, in a world we know is filled with fakers,
demagogues and "make believe" people, I thank my

Higher Power for what little I know, the understanding
God has given me, and the many blessings with which
God has showered me.

If I were to believe what little success I have
had was accomplished because of my own personal
knowledge or good judgment, I would be assuming too
much.

I want to be myself, an individual. It doesn't
matter how little I know, the fact that "Something"
helps me is all that matters.

126.   A POSITIVE ATTITUDE

"Life's a bitch and then you die." How many
times have I heard *that* one at meetings? I think that
in recovery, as well as in life, we get what we go after.

I remember hearing a woman compare main-
taining a positive mental attitude to putting wax on the
runners of a sled. It doesn't guide the sled down the hill
or navigate around obstacles, but it makes the ride
smoother and a lot more fun. That's what a positive
attitude in recovery can do, too.

Sure, recovery isn't always fun or without
pain; nothing worthwhile is. Having a negative outlook, though, encourages me to wallow in self-pity,
makes me forget the blessings I've already received,
and worse, lets me think I'm the absolute center of the

universe. Uh-uh. That's an old and dangerous tape for me.

I have a very short memory and need people around to remind me of what I want from the Program. I need to stay around the laughers, the positive thinkers, the winners. I don't want my life to be a bitch, and it doesn't have to be. It's my choice. A positive attitude is the right road for me, and staying positive *about* recovery makes the journey smoother and a lot more fun.

127.   SINGLE AND SEXY

There is a problem not often discussed around the meeting rooms. Nevertheless, it is a problem.

When drinking, we sometimes lacked morality. The song, *"All the Girls Get Prettier at Closing Time"* was a fact. With alcohol or drugs removing our inhibitions, it was easy to become involved in affairs or relationships.

Today, we are clean and sober. There are many divorced people in the Program as a result of their addiction. There is also an influx of young, single people coming to the Program due to an acute awareness of chemical dependency.

We are physically, morally, and spiritually bankrupt when we come to the Program. It is necessary to remove the guilt feelings of the past by *"Admitt[ing] to God, to ourselves, and to another human being, the exact nature of our wrongs."*

We must then continue to take a personal inventory and improve our conscious contact with God as we understand Him. Only then, *well past our first year of recovery,* may we hope to make any major changes in our lives. We must always remember that our primary purpose is to stay abstinent. Only when we work the Program are we useful.

By working the Steps of the Program and adhering to the principles, we find ourselves getting better. Feelings and emotions begin to return. An honest look within ourselves finds sexual yearning again rising.

A dilemma arises. What should one do? Most meetings are mixed and many friendly relationships can occur. A love and trust is built up between two people in the Program. To destroy this trust can be catastrophic to either or both parties. A relapse could be in the making.

The answers don't come easy. Individually, we have to decide for ourselves what we must do. The easiest, softest way I've heard is to go get drunk and pick up one of those people at closing time. But this is *not* the answer. On the other hand, there is difficulty involved with complete celibacy, although this works for some. For most of us, who realize that we are not saints, we stand at a turning point.

Because it is a personal decision, we find that going back to the "Four Absolutes" could give us a guide. Enter the relationship with complete *honesty*. Desires and motives must be absolutely *unselfish*. We must decide if our *love* is emotional or physical. If it is physical, forget it. The *purity* of our intentions must be examined. These decisions must be made with guidance from our Higher Power.

There is no pat answer. Serious consideration should be given to any relationship. The wrong decision can affect not only ourselves, but our friends and our group. The Absolutes can be extremely helpful when we want to do the right thing and the answer is not obvious.

When our recovery has a foundation firm enough to withstand stress, then we are ready to live, and love, in God's light.

128.   HONEST SHARING

Recently, our women's group invited a speaker, who came and shared with us honestly. Some people were thrilled, some were offended, some were neutral. But whether we liked what that speaker said or not, we were treated with truth.

That to me is what makes this Program special. Not too many masks can be worn when truth-hungry eyes are watching.

To our Fellowship's honest, soul-baring women speakers, I say: My hat is off to you, because of your courage in honestly telling what it was like, what happened, and what it is like now.

129.   HANDLING TENSION

Are you under constant strain because of "too much to do and too little time to do it"?

Stress and tension seem to be a part of modern living, with too much to be done, no time to relax, and everybody in a hurry. Here are some simple rules given by doctors to help ease your tensions, or at least, help you live with them.

Do one thing at a time. This is how to work your way out from under a load that seems too heavy. When you are tense, even ordinary jobs seem too much to handle.

Do the most urgent jobs one at a time, forgetting about the rest until later. Once these are finished, things won't look so bad and the other tasks will go more easily.

If you feel nothing can wait until later, you had better stop and reconsider. Are you sure you aren't giving too much importance to the things you do? Perhaps you think you are too important. Nobody is totally indispensable, so take it easy!

Don't set impossible goals for yourself. The Superwoman urge, the desire to be perfect in everything, causes worry and anxiety. Wherever you are going or whatever you are doing, start in time so you won't have to hurry.

Learn how to say "no" and when to say "yes." Because our time is limited, we need to learn to put first things first. Don't try to do it all.

Decide, too, which things you do well and put your major effort into these. As for the others, don't get upset if the job isn't perfect.

Life, in spite of its responsibilities, is to be enjoyed, so have some good times!

130. IT'S A.A., NOT AAA

When I first came into the Fellowship, I used the Program for emergencies only. I would wait until there was some sort of crisis, then I would try to put one of the principles into practice. The bulk of the time I did little to further my Program. Only when I was truly desperate did I work the Program.

Needless to say, I had several narrow escapes from the bottle. Ultimately, however, the time came when I had waited too long to try to correct a situation and I was too upset and thirsty to want to maintain my sobriety. I'd reached a point of no return. My habit of A.A. "for emergencies only" failed me and I was drunk again.

Since that time I have realized that the A.A. principles are better practiced every day, instead of once in a while. I believe that if the Program is practiced on a daily basis and a certain spiritual attitude is maintained, emergencies will be avoided.

When trying circumstances present themselves, we will have a spiritual reserve to call upon for the additional strength that's needed. As it says in the Big Book, *"It is easy to let up on the spiritual program of action and rest on our laurels. We are headed for trouble if we do, for alcohol is a subtle foe. We are not cured of alcoholism. What we really have is a daily reprieve contingent on the maintenance of our spiritual condition."*

Or, in the words of a good friend of mine, "A.A. is for maintenance; AAA is for emergencies!"

131. WHO IS RESPONSIBLE FOR WHAT?

I am the oldest of three kids. When I was 11, my brother 6, and my sister 2, my mother went into a tuberculosis sanitarium for the next seven years of our lives. I learned responsibility early, but think I may have gotten the wrong message.

We had a part-time housekeeper, but taking care of those kids became my responsibility most of the time.

My sister and a couple of little friends (about 7 years old) went on a shoplifting spree, and it was my fault because she was my responsibility.

My brother (about 12 years old) went rafting with friends down the Wisconsin River, and the fire department had to rescue them. It was my fault, because he was my responsibility.

What I am trying to say is that I was a responsible person but only where other people were concerned. I got so that I felt responsible for your feelings, actions, reactions, etc., and assumed responsibility where I had none.

What I never learned was to be responsible for myself. Oh sure, I worked so I could eat, buy clothes and pay for a roof over my head. But I never accepted responsibility for my own actions. As I had been responsible for other people, other people were responsible for me.

Then I learned in early recovery that "they" were not responsible for my actions, and I quickly grabbed onto the idea that "my addictions" did it all. There is no doubt that most of my bizarre, tacky, sleazy, etc., behavior was done under the influence, but not all of it. Today, I try not to take responsibility that is not mine, and to assume the responsibility that is mine alone. I am responsible for my own feelings and behavior; and I have to quit looking for other people, places, and situations to blame. The buck stops here!

132.   SEX: NOT A CURE
(13th Step)

The 13th Step is taken by people who suffer from the delusion that sex can cure their addiction. Women as well as men suffer from this malady. They're not always easy to spot. Some go to meetings and try to work the Program while others just sit around the clubs, eyeballing members of the opposite gender (usually newcomers), waiting for their chance to pounce. The newcomers, being somewhat bewildered, sometimes confuse lust with love and fall victim to this dangerous game.

John was an oldtimer. He'd managed to stay clean and sober (or dry, depending on who was taking his inventory) for ten years. His run-riot sexual desire had not been taken from him, however; and he believed that every willing woman was fair game.

Mary came into the Fellowship and met John. Mary was very pretty, and John offered to help her. Mary had been looking for a Higher Power and a Prince Charming all her life, and in her state of confusion, decided John was both.

Before long, Mary became too busy "being in love" with John to work her Program. She started trading 12-Step meetings for meetings with John. And it came to pass that Mary relapsed and couldn't understand why.

But John understood. He told everybody at his club (especially the young, female newcomers) that if Mary had worked the Program the way he did, she wouldn't have relapsed. And all the young, female newcomers held onto his every word, especially Jane, and John offered to help Jane....

Sex has never cured anyone's obsessions or addictions! When the "winners" say not to get "emotionally involved" with someone of the opposite sex for the first year of recovery, pay attention! The 13th Step could be very unlucky.

133.   TO LET GO

Does not mean I stop caring.
Is to care about, not care for.
Is not to change or blame others.
Is not to judge.
Is not to regret the past but to live and grow for the future.
Means to fear less, and love more.
And Let God!

134.   BUT CLOUDS GOT IN THE WAY

A fellow member asked for a ride home after our regular Tuesday night meeting. As we left the meeting she gazed into the sky and mentioned that she did not see the moon. I looked up and said that I did not see the stars and added that perhaps they were hidden by the clouds.

As we traveled toward her destination, we talked about the topic that she had brought up at the meeting. We discussed our reactions, present and past, to conditions similar to her present situation. As we discussed the topic, I became aware that my companion was beginning to relax. She began to slow down and started to weigh all facets of her situation. As she related some of the details of her problem to me, I could tell that her attitude toward the situation was changing and her problems did not seem to be so grim.

When we reached her destination, I looked up into the sky and noticed that the stars were brightly shining. Oddly enough, they had always been there; but I could not see them for the clouds.

The answers to my fellow member's problems were there, just as the stars and the moon; but she could not see them until she got the clouds out of the way.

So it is with our addiction, stinking thinking,

hate, anger, resentment, dishonesty, and a host of other traits. They are the clouds that blur and hide the answers that we need for a life of serenity, peace of mind, and happiness.

135. I MUST GO SHOPPING

I must go shopping. I am completely out of generosity and want to get some. I also want to exchange the self-satisfaction that I picked up the other day for some real humility; they say it wears better.

I want to look for tolerance, which is worn as a wrap this season. I saw some samples of kindness, and I'm a little low on that right now; one can't get too much of it.

I must try to match some patience. I saw it on a friend and it was so becoming. I must remember to get my sense of humor mended and keep my eyes open for inexpensive goodness.

Yes, I must go shopping today.

136. I HATE A.A.

When I hear such phrases as "alive again," "reborn," "a second chance to live," and others in a similar vein, I wonder what they mean to the speaker.

They form just one of the aspects of A.A. with which I find I cannot identify.

I am a simple soul. My opening remarks are merely an admission that I do not understand. There is nothing at all unusual in this, for there is little of the Program which I do understand. Yet it has worked for me for a considerable number of years, in spite of my lack of understanding, which would seem to indicate that *for me* acceptance may be of greater importance than understanding. For example, I do not understand when I hear people speak of their love for the Program. Personally, I hate it. Every Step, every Tradition, ever Concept of Service is diametrically opposed to my natural instincts. So to say that I love the Program would be to lie. However, I accept that it has to become an integral part of my life if I am to maintain my sobriety.

Before A.A. breathed the breath of life into me, I had wandered through this vale of tears seeing nothing which was real, hearing nothing which mattered, smelling nothing but the stench of my own corrupt decomposition, tasting nothing but the dregs of existence, and putting the mark of Cain on everything with which I came into contact. Only by the Grace of God, working through the Fellowship of A.A., did I start to live, *not again*, but for the first time.

I remember the amazement and joy of hearing, for the first time, the song of a bird. For the thirty-eight years prior to that evening, birds had been singing, but not for me. As I walked up the drive of that mental hospital, on my way to a meeting, it was as if that bird sang for me alone, sharing with me the joy of living, which I was beginning to experience for the first time.

Every worthwhile "first" has come with the growth of sobriety. The first time I knew the love and joy of holding a baby, it was not one of my five children, but when I held my first granddaughter. That was the first time I experienced the need to recognize the fragility of human beings, because there was no way I could hold that baby until I knew exactly how it should be done so that she would feel secure and free from fear.

I thank God for A.A. and thank you, the members of A.A., for teaching me that life is possible, and enjoyable, even for one who did not even know that life existed.

137.   HUMILITY PRAYER

Lord, I am far too much influenced by what people think of me.

Which means that I am always pretending to be either richer or smarter or nicer than I really am.

Please prevent me from trying to attract attention.

Don't let me gloat over praise on the one hand or be discouraged by criticism on the other.

Nor let me waste time weaving imaginary situations in which the most heroic, charming, witty person present is myself.

Show me how to be humble of heart like You.

138. NO FREE RIDE TO SPIRITUALITY

There is one oldtimer in A.A. who used to say things like "spirituality will get you drunk," and "God won't keep you sober," and I would argue and say, "Don't you know this is a spiritual program?" and "Haven't you ever read the ABC's which say *'No human power could relieve my alcoholism, and God could and would if He were sought'*?" He made me so mad. After a lot of time and much painful experience, I have to admit the old boy was right. I didn't realize it at the time, but my idea of "spirituality" had a lot of "magic" in it. I was seeking that great illuminating experience that would suddenly transform me into a new person. In other words, I wanted a FREE RIDE.

Not really being willing to "trudge that road of happy destiny," I wanted to be whisked effortlessly to my destination.

It is certain that God never knocked a drink out of my hand, and neither has He put a drink in my hand. What He *has* done is to give me a set of principles to live by, and a blessed Fellowship to share it with. I cannot get well in isolation, and I am perfectly capable of going to meetings seven nights a week and still stay in isolation. If I am not willing to get out of SELF by reaching out to you, then even God can't help me. If I can't come up with enough honesty to tell you how it really is with me, then I block God out of my life by my own pride. If I am not willing to apply the tools I have been given on a day-by-day, or sometimes minute-by-minute basis, then truly "God will not keep me sober."

So it appears that I am responsible for my own recovery; God is not. He has already done His part. Surely God stands ready to guide and strengthen if I will do my part. Part of me would much prefer to be a victim of circumstances. It's just a whole lot easier. The only problem is that continuing to be a victim will kill me. Today I love life (most of the time), and my desire is to live it to the maximum. I personally believe that A.A. and the 12 Steps represent the best recipe for good living ever created, but there are no "Free Rides." I have to DO IT.

139.   BECAUSE YOU SAID A PRAYER FOR ME

Because you said a prayer for me,
My view of life is brighter;
The darkness seemed to fade away,
And burdens grew much lighter.

Because you took the time to pray
A prayer for me today,
My tears were turned to laughter,
And joy returned to stay.

The world is full of hurt today,
And hearts are filled with care;
But many lives can still be touched
Because you said a prayer.

Thank you for caring.

140.   WHAT IS A SPONSOR?

A sponsor is someone you call on the telephone to tell her you are not speaking to her, and she listens to every word you are not saying.

A sponsor is the person you most fear to lose, so you tell her you don't want to see her; and she still comes when you call.

She accepts your insanity when you won't even admit it.

She knows you're only human when you're being God and judging her.

She remembers what you did when you had amnesia, and she still wants to know you.

She is responsible enough to care, but humble enough to know which decisions are yours, or God's.

She stands by her other commitments as well as you, so you call her selfish.

She is a tower of strength and a frail fragment of humanity. She gets her rotten days; do you share your good ones?

She is an alcoholic, too.

141. THE POWER OF PRAYER AND TRUST

In 1983 my husband called a treatment center and asked, "What is your success rate for atheists?" "The same as for believers," they replied. Later they told me, "It's often easier for you."

I quote this because I tried A.A. for varying periods between 1960 and 1980, but could not stay sober. Then it dawned on me that perhaps the one thing I had decided was "not for me," namely, a Higher

Power, was the secret to sobriety and recovery. I discovered that knowing and believing were two different things. How I envied tales of "flashes of enlightenment." It was necessary for me to work slowly to find a Higher Power.

I felt repeatedly lost, wondering whether the decisions I was making were right, continually feeling alone, until I was finally humble enough to catch myself praying, "I can't manage my own life. I have a long history of disasters. What is it You want to do with my life? I am willing to do what You want."

It took me a long time to reach that point. Looking back, I realize now I was being nudged in the right direction from the meetings I attended. Just as I had a compulsion to drink, I now had a compulsion to keep sober, and with it, a compulsion to believe in a Higher Power. That much I had on leaving the treatment center.

But how could I believe through this day-to-day living, clearing up the mess, getting a job, knowing and liking myself as I really am? Memory is not always our best friend; and I hope I do not exaggerate when I think back on those nights looking at the ceiling, sweating, walking around and around in panic, drinking cups of tea, smoking cigarettes, endlessly saying, "Please tell me what to do."

For someone taught to analyze and think for myself, developing trust and acceptance was very difficult. My monitoring system made me realize that every time I had courage to trust my Higher Power I seemed to make progress, not in material circumstances, but within myself. I had moments of peace and a reassurance that I was still on the muddy path that was leading to a firm concrete road; and that if I kept up the struggle, I would reach that road.

I cannot tell you how excited I was about that peace and reassurance. The dependency in me wanted to know who was in charge, but I knew I could only develop the relationship with prayer and trust, and by *not forgetting*.

For anyone who may be reading this and feeling lost, keep on working at it. I find that how I feel inside transcends everything in this day-to-day world, and how I feel depends on how I believe. For me, there is no sobriety or recovery without my Higher Power.

142.   DON'T QUIT

When things go wrong, as they sometimes will,
When the road you're trudging seems all uphill,
When the funds are low, and the debts are high,
And you want to smile, but you have to sigh,
When care is pressing you down a bit,
Rest if you must; but don't you quit.

Life is queer with its twists and turns,
As every one of us sometimes learns.
And many a failure turns about,
When she might have won had she stuck it out.
Don't give up though the pace seems slow;
You may succeed with another blow.

Success is failure turned inside out,
The silver tint of the clouds of doubt.
And you never can tell how close you are;
It may be near when it seems so far.
So stick to the fight when you're hardest hit;
It's when things seem worse
That you must not quit.

143. STRUGGLING FOR SOBRIETY
(13th Step)

I am a young female member of A.A., and I
have been in the Fellowship for a little over a year now.
I've been sad and lonely since I stopped drinking and
have been trying to overcome my feelings in my early
stages of growing up; I'm still a bit mixed up. And I
have some extra problems with which to cope.

First, I've had a few of the male A.A. members trying to get me to have sex with them; and
although one or two realize how much that has dis-

turbed me, they don't seem capable of understanding that when I say no, I mean NO. They don't seem to understand, or care, that I have a very good reason for saying no. I just do not want sex with them.

It's not that I'm a lesbian or anti-men; it's just that I've changed a lot since I put down the bottle and came to A.A. I've been trying so hard to make a decent life for myself and not "sleep around" any more. Before I came to A.A., I had been used and abused and hurt for far too long; now I'm struggling for sobriety, and that is difficult enough without having to cope with male members pestering me to get at my body. It not only prevents my progress, but increases my fear and anger, two things I have to get rid of or I will pick up a drink and die (or worse).

Another difficulty is trying to cope with unreliability. On one particular occasion, after successfully resisting repeated efforts to get at my body, we parted on good terms. I am basically a friendly, loving person, and perhaps a little stupid. I phoned him the next day to make sure we were still going to an A.A. function (we had made plans before the previous day), and he assured me we would still go. But he didn't turn up for me. I felt so let down.

As if all this were not enough, one member has been scheming more than the others, trying to seduce me away from my better way of life that I'm gradually building with the help of the A.A. Program and two caring sponsors. This man has been talking to me in a sly way, trying to get me to reveal intimate details of my past. But what really frightened me was when he told me that alcohol would not affect me now!

Fortunately for me, I'm not that stupid. I know very well what booze will do, and I want none of it. I want to stay away from alcohol and get well and live a sober life.

If these people want to get sober and not stay one of the "un-drunks," I suggest they start examining themselves. They may need help to solve their problems, but help is available if they seek it.

But what about me? How can I make progress and get a little serenity?

144.   12 RULES NOT TO LIVE BY

1.   It is a dire necessity to be loved and approved of by every significant person in my life.

2.   I should be thoroughly competent, adequate, and achieving in all possible aspects.

3.   Some people are bad, wicked, or vile and should (or must be) punished.

4.   If things do not go (or stay) the way I very much want them to, it would be awful, catastrophic, or terrible.

5.   Unhappiness is externally caused, and I can-

not control it (unless I control the other person).

6. One should remain upset or worried if faced with a dangerous or fearsome reality.

7. It is easier to avoid responsibility and difficulties than to face them.

8. I have a right to be dependent and people (or someone) should be strong enough to rely on (or take care of me).

9. My early childhood experiences must continue to control me and determine my emotions and behavior.

10. I should become upset over my and other people's problems or behavior.

11. There is invariably one right, precise, and perfect solution; and it would be terrible and catastrophic if this solution is not found.

12. The world (and especially other people) should be fair, and justice (or mercy) must triumph.

145. MY SIDEKICK

My "sidekick" is with me most of the time. I'd like to call her my friend, but I've really come to know the loneliness and despair she's caused.

Funny, but since she's been around so long I would have thought I would have gotten to know her better and recognize her traits and understand why I've allowed her around so long. You see, she's really not all bad; she's helped me many, many times to avoid people, to not allow people to hurt me, to shield me from rejection.

It was so gradual I didn't really notice it, but I began to turn to her more and more in the last few years. When I didn't want to be with other people, when I was depressed, when I was angry or frustrated or bitter, or whatever, she was always there to encourage me.

Then a strange thing happened. I began to fear she was the only friend I would have left one day, because I was so dependent on her. She seemed intelligent and supplied all the self-pity I wanted. She seemed to know when to join me and when to stay away. She was so sympathetic; it was like she could take me out of every situation and every place into an existence of despair and loneliness.

Everyone else was always to blame. She let me know along the way that there was something wrong with all those other people for not wanting to associate with me or be friendly or even just talk.

She knows about my addictions; and even though early in recovery I realized I was allowing her to use me for her purposes and understood I shouldn't associate with her any more, I allowed her to come around because it was comfortable. I hadn't ever really invited her to join me in the first place; but when I began to get somewhat well in recovery, I began to be friendlier with other people and not so withdrawn. Every time I let myself go, she would come back automatically; and there I would be in a crowd with her, and no one really even noticed me.

I felt as if I really wasn't there! You see, I thought others felt uncomfortable with her around. In reality, it was the awareness of the goodness in others, in myself, and that God is always with me that prompted me to ask my Higher Power to take her out of my life.

I also experienced a lot of pain in letting go of her, but it had to be done, for she stood in the way of my love for myself and others, and in my fullness to receive God. The Program has taught me so much; for instance, a continuing effort to be willing to let go and to accept.

I suppose it's time I revealed her name: it's "Isolation."

Since this inner revelation, I have learned that Isolation is not all bad, perhaps not at all. There are times that she is still with me, but I have come to know her in another way. She listens quietly as I meditate and pray and talk with God! I suppose I could say she's merged into being a part of my being in this growing process of recovery, thanks to the Program, the people in the Program, my sponsor, and my Higher Power, God!

146.   DECORATE YOUR OWN SOUL

After a while you learn the subtle difference between holding a hand and chaining a soul; and you learn that love doesn't mean owning and company doesn't always mean security; and you begin to learn that kisses aren't contracts and presents aren't promises; and you begin to accept your defeats with your head up and your eyes ahead with the grace of an adult, not the grief of a child.

You learn to build all your roads on today because tomorrow's ground is too uncertain for plans, and futures have a way of falling down in mid-flight. After a while you learn that even sunshine burns if you get too much.

So, you plant your own garden and decorate your own soul, instead of waiting for someone else to bring you flowers.

You learn that you really *can* endure, that you are strong, that you *do* have worth, that you *are* beautiful.

147.   THE STATION

Tucked away in our subconscious minds is an idyllic vision. We see ourselves on a long, long trip that almost spans the continent. We're traveling by passenger train, and out the windows we drink in the passing scene of cars on nearby highways, of children waving at a crossing, of cattle grazing on a distant hillside, of smoke pouring from a power plant, of row upon row of corn and wheat, of flatlands and valleys, of mountains and rolling hillsides, of city skylines and village hills, of biting winter and blazing summer and cavorting spring and docile fall.

But uppermost in our minds is the final destination. On a certain day at a certain hour, we will pull into the station. There will be bands playing and flags flying. And once we get there so many wonderful dreams will come true.

So many wishes will be fulfilled and so many pieces of our lives finally will be neatly fitted together like a completed jigsaw puzzle. How restlessly we pace the aisles, damning the minutes for loitering, waiting, waiting, waiting for the station.

However, sooner or later we must realize there is no one station, no one place to arrive at once and for all. The true joy of life is the trip. The station is only a dream. It constantly outdistances us.

"When we reach the station, that will be it!" we cry. Translated it means, "When I'm 18, that will be it! When I buy a new 450 SL Mercedes-Benz, that will be it! When I put the last kid through college, that will be it! When I have paid off the mortgage, that will be it! When I win a promotion, that will be it! When I reach the age of retirement, that will be it! I shall live happily ever after."

Unfortunately, once we get "it," then "it" disappears. The station somehow hides itself at the end of an endless track.

"Relish the moment" is a good motto, especially when coupled with Psalm 118:24: "This is the day which the Lord hath made; we will rejoice and be glad in it." It isn't the burdens of today that drive men mad. Rather, it is regret over yesterday or fear of tomorrow. Regret and fear are twin thieves who would rob us of today.

So stop pacing the aisles and counting the miles. Life must be lived as we go along. The station will come soon enough.

148. STINKING THINKING

A brand-new member who had wholeheartedly accepted the Program was busily telling me that now she would be able to work harder, pay off her bills, move to a better place, get a car of her own, etc.

I repeated to her our God-given slogan, "Easy Does It," several times, but the onrush of "now I can do this," continued. Then I heard myself saying, "Don't forget; you can't brush your teeth and tie your shoelaces at the same time."

She fell silent for a minute, then said, "Thanks, that straightened that out. As you said, do one thing at a time and take one day at a time."

The somewhat ludicrous mental image of a person crouching over a washbowl with a toothbrush at a jaunty angle in the mouth, while fumbling blindly for unseen shoelaces, has a sobering effect on us. We alcoholics have spent a life running madly off in all directions to do all things at once, with, of course, no real accomplishment. The phrase reduces our inner turmoil and anxiety to its simplest terms in a comical manner that makes it stick.

"Easy does it," "One day at a time," "Accept the things I cannot change," "Change the things I can," all are simple statements. Yet, to us, with our susceptibility to "stinking thinking," how difficult sometimes to comprehend. How easy it is for us to be thrown by some temporary problem, or setback, that requires a cool, calm, immediate handling, without the handicap of a liquor-soaked mind.

The image of the fool with his head in a washbowl, fumbling blindly for unseen shoelaces, has served me well. The face in the washbowl can quickly become the face at the bar.

And "you can't brush your teeth and tie your shoelaces at the same time" has helped me handle daily problems with a smile, at least for the one day at a time with which I have been blessed.

149. FROM A NEWCOMER

You were the first person to reach out to me. With honesty, sincerity, understanding, and compassion, there you were for me. Many people relate to me in many different ways, and on many different levels, but few can understand and read me as you do. And in your special way you let me know that, in those first few days of my sobriety. Through your sharing, I came to understand that I was not so unique after all, but that I did belong, that I could recover. You accepted me unequivocally, and you inspired me to continue on in this Program. To you I am so very grateful. For your quality sobriety, your dedication, your willingness, your openmindedness, and your honesty, and for those three little words you first spoke to me, "so am I," I thank you and applaud you.

150. RECOVERY

Recovery is the most important thing in your life, without exception. You may believe your job, or your home life, or one of many other things, comes first. But consider: if you don't stay with the Program, chances are you won't have a job, a family, sanity, or even life. If you are convinced that everything in life depends on your recovery, you have a much better chance of improving your life. If you put other things first, you are only hurting your chances.

IT
WORKS
IT REALLY
DOES

THE TWELVE STEPS

1. We admitted we were powerless over alcohol that our lives had become unmanageable.
2. Came to believe that a Power greater than ourselves could restore us to sanity.
3. Made a decision to turn our will and our lives over to the care of God *as we understood Him*.
4. Made a searching and fearless moral inventory of ourselves.
5. Admitted to God, to ourselves, and to another human being the exact nature of our wrongs.
6. Were entirely ready to have God remove all these defects of character.
7. Humbly asked Him to remove our shortcomings.
8. Made a list of all persons we had harmed, and became willing to make amends to them all.
9. Made direct amends to such people wherever possible, except when to do so would injure them or others.
10. Continued to take personal inventory and when we were wrong promptly admitted it.
11. Sought through prayer and meditation to improve our conscious contact with God *as we understood Him*, praying only for knowledge of His will for us and the power to carry that out.
12. Having had a spiritual awakening as the result of these steps, we tried to carry this message to alcoholics, and to practice these principles in all our affairs.

The Twelve Steps are reprinted with permission of A.A. World Services, Inc., New York, New York.

PHONE NUMBERS AND NOTES

_____

_____

_____

_____

_____

_____

_____

_____

_____

_____

_____

_____

_____

PHONE NUMBERS AND NOTES

_____

_____

_____

_____

_____

_____

_____

_____

_____

_____

_____

_____

_____

PHONE NUMBERS AND NOTES

_____

_____

_____

_____

_____

_____

_____

_____

_____

_____

_____

_____

_____

PHONE NUMBERS AND NOTES

_____

_____

_____

_____

_____

_____

_____

_____

_____

_____

_____

_____

PHONE NUMBERS AND NOTES

PHONE NUMBERS AND NOTES

_____

_____

_____

_____

_____

_____

_____

_____

_____

_____

_____

_____

PHONE NUMBERS AND NOTES

PHONE NUMBERS AND NOTES

PHONE NUMBERS AND NOTES

Inquiries, orders, and catalog requests
should be addressed to:

Glen Abbey Books, Inc.
P.O. Box 31329
Seattle, Washington 98103
Call toll-free (all U.S.) 1-800-782-2239